SCALE
BACK!

SCALE
BACK!

WHY CHILDHOOD OBESITY IS NOT JUST ABOUT WEIGHT

WILLOW INTERNATIONAL LIBRARY

Kathi A. Earles, M.D., M.P.H.
and Sandra E. Moore, M.D.

Edited by Cynthia Thomas

HILTON PUBLISHING COMPANY

Hilton Publishing Company
Chicago, IL

Direct all correspondence to:
Hilton Publishing Company
1630 45th Street, Suite 103
Munster, IN 46321
219–922–4868
www.hiltonpub.com

Notice: The information in this book is true and complete to the best of the authors' knowledge. This book is intended only as an information reference and should not replace, countermand, or conflict with the advice given to readers by their physicians. The authors and publisher disclaim all liability in connection with the specific personal use of any and all information provided in this book.

Library of Congress Cataloging-in-Publication Data

Earles, Kathi, 1963-
   Scale back! : why childhood obesity is not just about weight / Kathi A. Earles, Sandra E. Moore.
     p. cm.
     ISBN 0–9743144–8–X
   1. Obesity in children. I. Moore, Sandra E., 1973- II. Title.
RJ399.C6E268 2007   618.92'398—dc22
                                           2007048899

Printed and bound in the United States of America

CONTENTS

ACKNOWLEDGMENTS

Dr. Earles' Acknowledgments

Thank you Jordan, Riley, and Jax for giving me lots of cuddle time, kisses, and endless humor. Thank you Allie for being my husband, boyfriend, and best friend all rolled into one. I love you family.

The authors wish to thank Drs. Najaz Woods, Yvonne Fry-Johnson, and Yasmin Tyler-Hill for their contributions to *Scale Back*. We appreciate you.

Dr. Moore's Acknowledgments

This book is dedicated to all children who suffer with weight problems and all parents who are struggling with this issue. I dedicate this book to my community in the hopes it will increase health, nutrition, and well being for everyone. I would like to thank my mother, Elizabeth, for all her love and support, and my sister, Cynthia, for being my sounding board.

PREFACE

The most important thing we can do for our children is to raise them in a happy and healthy environment. As a parent, you know whether or not your children are truly happy: Do they get along with other children? Do they have a lot of friends? Are they participating in activities they enjoy? All parents have a common goal for their children—that they grow up strong, successful, happy, and healthy.

As pediatricians, we are seeing more and more overweight and obese children. In fact, overweight and its more dangerous counterpart, obesity, have become national problems affecting both children and adults. We are concerned about "overweight" and "obesity" because of the diseases such as stroke, high blood pressure, and heart disease that are associated with excess weight and inactivity. As healthcare providers, we want children to thrive. Preventing disease and maintaining health are top priorities for pediatricians; we give children vaccines to prevent diseases such as polio and measles; we stress the importance of seat belts while riding in cars and helmets while riding bikes to minimize injuries from accidents. Childhood obesity should be viewed in the same way. Our goal is to *prevent* the health problems caused, and worsened, by excessive weight. Teaching our children good dietary and fitness habits early in life can reduce the likelihood that they will gain excessive weight as adults. As we all know, the habits formed in childhood are more easily carried over into adulthood.

This book will discuss the many facets of childhood overweight and obesity. It is our aim to help you understand the problem and, as importantly, how to deal with it. Because we know that overweight doesn't only affect children, but often affects the entire family, we have included some useful information for parents. Armed with this knowledge, you can help your children develop good dietary and exercise habits to stay healthy and fit as they grow into adulthood. We encourage you to live by example and make healthy habits a "family affair."

CHAPTER ONE

What Size Is Right?

Objectives

- Become familiar with the trend towards overweight in children
- Understand the role race and ethnicity play in overweight trends
- Understand factors that have contributed to overweight in children
- Learn what is considered a "healthy" size for children
- Learn how to determine if your child is overweight

Overweight Trends in Children: The Bare Facts

If you read the newspapers or turn on the TV, you have probably heard about the "Obesity Epidemic." Lately, it seems as if everywhere you turn "experts" are talking of this new problem that Americans face—obesity. But when you look at your family and community, do you think people have really gotten bigger or is this all just hype? As you remember back to your school days, how do today's children measure up to you and your childhood friends? While most of us were considered "average" sized kids, being "chubby" was not uncommon, but in the last thirty years the rate of childhood overweight in the U.S. has tripled, jumping from roughly 5% to 15%. Let's take a look at what has happened to American children over the past thirty years.

Using the largest database of children's heights and weights, we have learned a lot about childhood obesity. Between 1971 and 1974, only 4% of 6–11 year olds were considered overweight. By 2004, that number jumped to 18.8%. Similarly, between 1971 and 1974, just 8% of 12–19 year olds were overweight, but in 2004, that number rose to 17.4%. (See Figure 1.)

The evidence is clear—overall, the frequency of overweight has increased dramatically for children and teenagers. Furthermore, overweight is even a bigger problem depending upon gender and ethnicity. Figure 2 shows that for Black girls ages 12–19, the rate of overweight is 25.4%, compared to 15.4% of White girls and 14.1% of Mexican girls. For girls younger than twelve, 26.5% of Black girls are overweight compared to 17% of White girls and 19% of Mexican girls. Among boys 12 -19, the rate of overweight is pretty much the same for Blacks, Whites, and Mexicans, about 18.5%. Among the younger boys, 25% of Mexican boys are overweight compared to 18.5% and 17.5% percent of White and Black boys respectively. Data for other ethnic groups have not been collected as consistently, but some data indicate that overweight among Native American children in the Southwestern United States is as high as 40%.

In practice, many parents ask how do we know this information or from where does it derive? These are very good questions: Let us try to explain. The Centers for Disease Control and

FIGURE 1.1

Overweight Trends in Children Over the Past 30 years

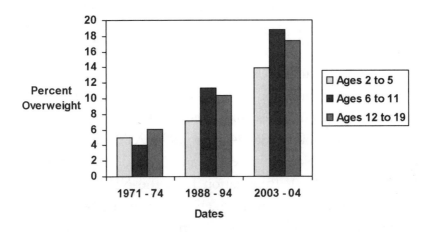

Source: www.cdc.gov

FIGURE 1.2

Prevalence of Overweight Among Children and Adolescents
Ages 6–19 Years

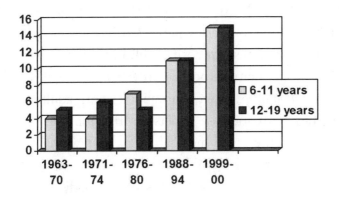

Source: aspe.hhs.gov

Prevention (CDC), is one of the nation's leading federal agencies that reports on disease and health statistics. The CDC periodically conducts studies of heights, weights, and other health indicators of specific groups of people in the United States. These studies include men, women, and children of varying ethnic groups, including African Americans, Caucasians, and Mexican Americans. The CDC has collected thousands of measurements at various times during the past forty years—1963–70, 1971–74, 1976–80, 1988–94, and 1999–2000. This study is known as the National Health and Nutrition Examination Survey (NHANES). Information from the NHANES surveys can be compared to see what the trends are in a given area. For our purposes, we looked at the national trends of overweight in children.

What is Overweight and Obesity?

You will hear the words **obese** and **overweight** often throughout this book and in the media when referring to the current crisis with U.S. children. But what is meant by "overweight?" What is meant by "obese?" Are the words interchangeable, or do they mean something different when referring to your child's weight? How do doctors determine if a child or adult is overweight or obese? For simplicity throughout this book, we will use the terms *overweight and obese* interchangeably for both adult and children since they both increase a person's risk for disease. Please be advised that these are medical terms and we caution parents NOT to refer to their child as obese or overweight as he or she may feel self-conscious about his or her body and may lose a sense of self-worth.

The Body Mass Index

Medically, doctors can determine whether a person is overweight or obese by using the Body Mass Index. The Body Mass Index (BMI) is a measurement scale that health professionals use to esti-mate the amount of excess weight in the body. The BMI has been used in studies that look for associations between weight and dis-eases such as diabetes and high blood pressure. As the BMI increases above a certain level, so does an individual's risk for the development of certain diseases. However, not everyone who has a high BMI is at risk. Very muscular people such as bodybuilders and highly trained athletes are the exception. Although these groups tend to weigh more, they also tend to have extra muscle weight, not fat. Therefore, for them, the BMI is not a reliable indi-cator of risk for disease. In fact, these people have much lower chances for developing diseases associated with overweight than the general population. We want to emphasize that this is the exception; the vast majority of us can use the BMI as an indicator of body fat and a predictor for disease development.

How to Calculate BMI

The body mass index is calculated the same way for adults and children, but the results are interpreted differently. The BMI is calculated using a person's height and weight. One formula for calculating the BMI is as follows:

BMI = Weight (in pounds) x 703 = X
Divide X by Height (in inches) = Y
Divide Y by Height (in inches) = BMI

An example of how to calculate BMI for a 5 foot 5 inches tall (65 inches) 140 lb. person is:

140 x 703= 98,420
98,420 ÷ 65 = 1,514.15
1,514.15 ÷ 65= 23.29
This person's BMI is 23.29

What do the numbers mean for adults?

For adults, cutoffs are used to establish if a person is *underweight*, *normal weight*, *overweight*, or *obese*. The following chart shows the standard interpretations for BMI measurements for adult men and women:

BMI	Weight Category
Below 18.5	Underweight
18.5–24.9	Normal Weight
25–29.9	Overweight
30.0 and above	Obese

As you can see, a BMI measurement above 25 is considered overweight and if the BMI rises to measurements above 30, a person is considered obese. All people, regardless of race or ethnicity, have a significantly increased risk for diseases at BMI measurements above 25, and an even greater risk at a BMI above 30.

Since children are constantly growing, we cannot use these absolute cutoffs. We must take into consideration a child's age and gender. (Certainly a three-year-old child should be smaller than a ten-year old, whom should be smaller than a seventeen-year old.) Once the BMI is calculated for a child, it is then plotted on a graph to compare the child to other children of the same age and gender. These are standard plotting graphs developed by the CDC. (See Figure 3, "BMI Chart for Girls," and Figure 4, "BMI Chart for Boys.")

What do the numbers mean for children?

Let's look at the BMI charts for boys and girls. First you will notice that there is a chart for girls, which is different from the chart for boys. This is because boys and girls have different growth patterns. Across the bottom of the chart, horizontally, you will see the *age*. Along the vertical sides of the chart you see "BMI". Swooping across the chart you see additional lines with a number near the end on the right (5, 10, 25, 50, 75, 85, 90, and 95). These numbers refer to *percentiles*. Percentile simply refers to the percentage of children whose BMI is less than that number. For example, if an eleven-year-old boy has a BMI of 19, then his BMI is at the 75th percentile. This means that his BMI is higher than 75% of all the eleven-year-old boys in the United States. Keep in mind:

- Children with a body mass index (BMI) between the 85th and 94th percentile are considered overweight.
- Children with a BMI greater than the 95th percentile (over the top line on the graph) are considered "obese."

Just like adults, overweight and obese children are at a higher risk for developing diseases associated with overweight compared

FIGURE 1.3

BMI Chart for Girls aged 2–20

2 to 20 years: Girls
Body mass index-for-age percentiles

NAME _____

RECORD # _____

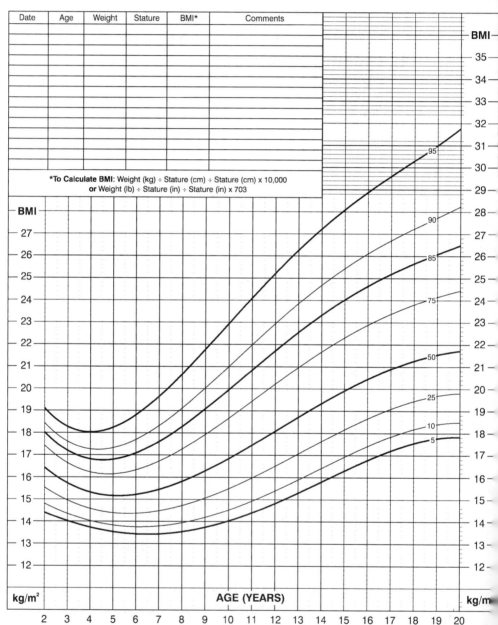

*To Calculate BMI: Weight (kg) ÷ Stature (cm) ÷ Stature (cm) x 10,000
or Weight (lb) ÷ Stature (in) ÷ Stature (in) x 703

Published May 30, 2000 (modified 10/16/00).
SOURCE: Developed by the National Center for Health Statistics in collaboration with
the National Center for Chronic Disease Prevention and Health Promotion (2000).
http://www.cdc.gov/growthcharts

SAFER • HEALTHIER • PEOPLE

FIGURE 1.4

BMI Chart for Boys aged 2–20

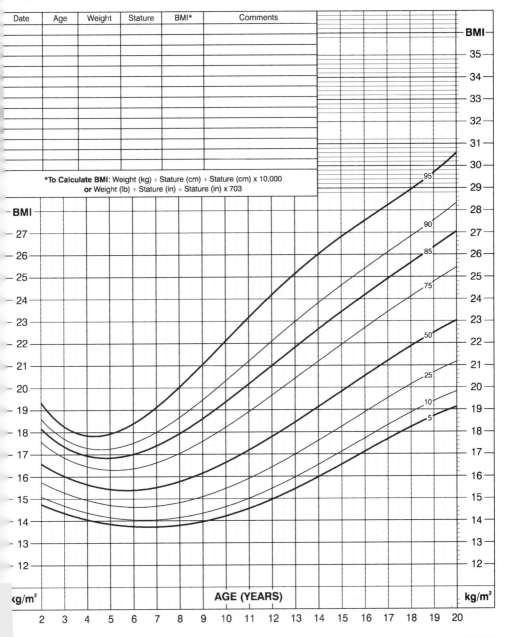

2 to 20 years: Boys
Body mass index-for-age percentiles

NAME _____

RECORD # _____

Date	Age	Weight	Stature	BMI*	Comments

*To Calculate BMI: Weight (kg) ÷ Stature (cm) ÷ Stature (cm) x 10,000
or Weight (lb) ÷ Stature (in) ÷ Stature (in) x 703

AGE (YEARS)

Published May 30, 2000 (modified 10/16/00).
SOURCE: Developed by the National Center for Health Statistics in collaboration with
the National Center for Chronic Disease Prevention and Health Promotion (2000).
http://www.cdc.gov/growthcharts

CDC
SAFER · HEALTHIER · PEOPLE

to normal weight children. And as is the case for adults, standard BMI charts for children apply to children of all races. Even if your child is obese according to his or her BMI, using a term like "extra weight" may be more appropriate when discussing this sensitive subject with your child.

Breaking Down the Difference in Overweight Trends: Genetics Versus Environment, Culture and Location

The rate of overweight in the United States differs not only between boys and girls, but also between African Americans, Caucasians, and Mexican Americans as displayed in Table 1.1. The differences between ethnic groups are due to many reasons.

Genetics

The first and most common belief is that the differences can be explained by genes. Genes are the genetic material passed on by parents to children; they determine all the characteristics of a person. For example, genes determine your eye and hair color, your blood type, and your height. Genes stay the same for a very long time in human populations. If you compared your genes to your great-great grandmother's you would find they are very similar.

Because genes stay pretty stable over very long periods of time, it is very unlikely to say that the changes we have seen in overweight trends in the past thirty years are due to genes alone. Some people may have genes which make them store extra energy. If your body can do this better than other people, then you will have more fat than other people (and possibly be over-

TABLE 1.1

Percent of Children Overweight in 1999–2000 by Age,
Gender and Race

		Total	African Americans	Mexican Americans	Caucasians
Boys	6–11	17	17	27	14
	12–19	17	19	25	15
Girls	6–11	15	23	17	13
	12–19	15	24	20	13

Source: www.cdc.gov

weight). But even if you have genes that are more likely to help you be overweight, you still have to eat too much food to gain excessive weight. Remember, your grandparents and great grandparents had your genes too, but many of them were not overweight, especially when they were children.

We have also heard some African Americans say that they are "big-boned," or have larger frames. While there can be some differences in body compositions among different ethnic groups—African Americans and Mexican Americans can have slightly larger bones and muscle—this difference is not enough to account for the major weight difference between them and other ethnic groups. So although genes can play an important role in determining how much you weigh, the bottom line is not everyone is "designed" to be the same size. But this fact should not limit us in our quest to promote healthy lifestyles for ourselves and our children.

Cultural Differences

Our cultural traditions may even be more important than our
genetic makeup. Our environment may also play a major role in
both adult and childhood obesity. One of the things which
make our country so great is all the different cultures we enjoy,
but some of our cultural norms may be contributing to the overweight trend. Weight is not viewed the same way by all ethnic
groups. Even individuals within the same culture do not view
weight in the same manner. We need to take a moment to recognize these differences. In some cultures, and especially in
mainstream American culture, being a thin woman or girl is
viewed as normal and there may be extreme pressure to be what
some may classify as "thin." We are bombarded on a daily basis
with the latest diet craze and images of what is portrayed as the
"perfect body." This need for body perfection has led countless
girls and women, and to a lesser extent, boys and men, to
develop eating disorders such as *anorexia nervosa* and *bulimia*.
(These weight-related conditions will be discussed in Chapter
4.) By contrast, some cultures regard "softer," "rounder" female
figures as being more desirable than "skinny" women or even
women of *normal* weight. They may in fact view normal weight
women as being *too* thin. Sometimes too in these cultures parents are more concerned with the health of their normal weight
children than with their overweight children. They may view a
normal weight child as thin, and therefore unhealthy, versus an
overweight child who may be viewed as "healthy." This notion
is more common in African-American and other ethnic communities. In fact, there are many myths concerning weight in
the African-American community. Some of the more common
ones are:

1. "I'm meant to be big. My whole family is big."
2. "I have big bones."
3. "There's no use in exercising. I can't exercise."
4. "I gain weight no matter what I eat."
5. "As long as I look good, my weight doesn't matter."

While we appreciate and celebrate cultural differences, they should not be used as barriers to emphasizing good nutrition and exercise habits for *all* people. Healthy bodies can be achieved with a balanced diet and daily physical activity, regardless of genetic makeup or cultural influences.

Economic Status

In addition to genes and culture, a person's economic status may also influence weight. Socioeconomic status refers to a person's level of income which allows him or her to afford housing, transportation, food, clothing, and other necessities. A person's socioeconomic status can define many aspects of life: Many people rarely associate their everyday routine with socioeconomic status, but where you live and the amount of money you earn can determine how healthy you are: Are the supermarkets in your neighborhood stocked with fresh fruits and vegetables? Or are there mostly packaged foods on the shelves? Is your neighborhood safe enough for you to exercise outside? Do the schools provide healthy lunches for your children, or do they serve the standard cafeteria fare? Do they have snack food vending machines? Do they offer exercise as a part of the daily curriculum?

The problems that these questions pose are not easily solved. Some people may be surprised to learn there are far fewer supermarkets in low-income areas than there are in more wealthy neighborhoods. In addition, these supermarkets are often over-priced and poorly stocked. The simple solution, some might say, would be for lower-income people to drive to the better-stocked supermarkets that have a greater variety of produce and may feature lower prices. Although this might seem to be a quick solution, many of these supermarkets are usually quite a distance from lower-income areas. Many families may not have a car or reliable transportation to make the trip. Low-income families also have other financial burdens that they need to consider and healthier food choices may not be a priority.

Lack of Physical Activity

Access to physical activity can also be a problem. Some neighborhoods may have few or no recreation centers or sports programs. Parents may feel the neighborhood is not safe enough for their children to play outdoors. As a result, these children are often confined to their homes to watch television or play video games, in essence becoming a "couch potato." Children living in wealthier neighborhoods often have access to recreational facilities, organized team sports, and family outings. Yet, despite these and other obstacles, making health a priority for your children and family can add years to their lives, so it is well worth your investment in time and effort to make some positive changes. Later in the book we will discuss options for healthy food-shopping and exercise activities you can perform indoors.

Underlying Medical Causes of Overweight in Children

Some people, including children, have medical problems which can cause them to become overweight. However, these cases are very rare. How quickly your body burns calories is referred to as your metabolism. Your metabolism depends on many factors, such as age, gender, activity level, and, of course, genes. Some people seem to burn calories very quickly, while others seem to use them very slowly. This can be true even within the same family. Weight can vary even among people who eat the same things. But even if your metabolism is slower than average, this fact alone should not cause a lot of weight gain. Often there are other reasons, like not eating properly and not exercising enough. This is especially true for children, who, because of their younger age and activity level, rarely have what is considered a slow metabolism.

In the majority of adults and children, overweight is caused by simply eating too much food and not getting enough exercise. If you think your child could have a medical problem as a cause of overweight, ask yourself the following questions:

1. Is my child shorter than other children of the same age and gender?
2. Is my child developmentally delayed? For example, does my child appear to have similar physical and mental skills as other children his or her age?
3. Does my child complain of excessive tiredness, or feeling cold all the time?
4. Did my child gain a lot of weight in a very short period of time?

If you answered yes to any of the above questions, you should check with your healthcare provider to make sure that your child does not have an underlying medical condition that could be the cause of excessive weight gain. Rarely, there can be hormonal or genetic problems that make a child overweight. We want to emphasize that these problems are not common and you should discuss any concerns you may have with your child's healthcare provider.

Summing It All Up

Overweight and obesity are growing problems among American youth and adults. There are many factors that contribute to childhood overweight, but an underlying medical condition is rarely the cause. Although genes may play a role, genes alone are not the main reason for the obesity epidemic. More importantly, our cultural and socioeconomic status influence our eating and activity habits. Understanding obesity, overweight, and your child's weight status is the first line of defense in fighting these problems.

CHAPTER 1 • EXERCISE A

Use the worksheet below to calculate the BMI for each member of your family. To complete this exercise, you will need a scale and tape measure. To begin, let us review how to take the measurements:

1. Record your child's weight *in pounds* from the scale.
2. Record the height in *inches*. If you do not know your child's height, hold a tape measure vertically to a flat

wall. Make sure it is straight and then tape it to the wall. Then have your child stand against the tape measure with a straight back.

3. Multiply the weight by 703.
4. Divide that answer by the height in inches.
5. Divide that answer again by the height in inches. The result is the BMI.

Weight in pounds	
Multiply by 703	
	Answer:
Divide answer by height in inches	
	Answer:
Divide answer again by height in inches	
	Result is your BMI:

For adults, circle the weight status that corresponds to your BMI result:

Less than 18.5	= underweight
Between 18.6 – 24.9	= ideal weight
Between 25 – 29.9	= overweight
Greater than 30	= obese

For children, plot the BMI on the appropriate growth chart to determine the percentile. If the child is female, use the chart in Figure 3. If the child is male, use the chart in Figure 4. Make sure you have plenty of copies of the growth charts for practice. Each child should be plotted on a separate graph. It can be tricky, so you may need to practice a number of times.

First look across the bottom of the chart and locate your child's age. If your child is between ages, use the most appropriate line closest to his or her age or somewhere in the middle of the two ages. For example if your child is 5 years and 6 months, go halfway between the 5 and the 6. If your child is 10 years, 3 months, go closer to 10 years. Once you have found your child's proper age, draw a line from that point to the top of the page. Next, go to the left or right hand side of the graph, where you will find BMI numbers. Locate your child's BMI number and draw a line to the other side of the paper. Where the two lines intersect is where your child "plots" on the graph.

Once you have plotted your child's BMI, see which of the percentile lines he or she is on. Some children may plot in-between lines. Write the percentile line your child BMI plots on, or if the plotted BMI lies between two percentile lines, write both numbers.

My child's BMI percentile lies on _____

OR

My child's BMI percentile is between _____ AND _____

Circle the weight status that corresponds to the number(s) on the lines above:

Less than 5th percentile	= underweight
Between 5th–84th percentile	= ideal weight
Between 85th-94th percentile	= overweight
Greater than 95th percentile	= obese

If your child is underweight, you should see your child's doctor to discuss his or her weight. Likewise if your child is overweight, with a BMI equal to or greater than the 85th percentile, he or she should also be evaluated by a physician.

CHAPTER 1 • EXERCISE B

In this exercise, place a checkmark next to any of the following statements that apply to you.

☐ My child's BMI is equal to or greater than the 85th percentile for his or her age and gender.

☐ I am overweight or obese and worry about my child having the same issue.

☐ I have immediate family members with high blood pressure, Type 2 diabetes, asthma, or joint problems associated with obesity.

☐ My child has unhealthy eating habits (eats large quantities of food or a lot of high calorie foods).

☐ My child gets little or no exercise.

☐ I worry that my child's weight is out of control.

☐ I am concerned about my child's health because of his or her weight.

If you answered yes to any of these questions, you should consult your child's doctor.

CHAPTER TWO

Healthy Eating for Everyone

Objectives

- Learn how calorie intake influences weight
- Learn the basic food units (fats, proteins, carbohydrates)
- Learn why fiber is necessary
- Learn the importance of vitamins and minerals
- Learn to make healthier choices
- Learn how to read food labels

If your child is overweight, you might be considering putting him or her on a diet. Rather than a quick-fix eating plan for weight loss, you should consider instead a lifestyle change that incorporates healthy eating and consistent exercise. To guide you on the path to a positive lifestyle change, we will help you understand what calories are and how the body uses them. We will also show you how carbohydrates, fats, and protein nourish the body and why fiber is important.

What Are Calories?

A calorie is a measure of energy expenditure. You may also see the word "kilocalorie" (kcal) in books and articles on nutrition, diet, or exercise. Simply put, one calorie or kilocalorie is equal to 3,500 units of food energy, which is equal to one pound of body weight. If you need to lose one pound, you will need to burn 3,500 units of energy.

We eat calories in the form of food and use or burn calories with every activity we perform. Calories come from fats, carbohydrates, and proteins. If you eat more calories than you use, you will gain weight. If you burn more calories than you eat, you will lose weight. If the calories you eat equal the calories you use, you will stay at the same weight. Pretty simple, huh? Well if it is so simple why do so many people struggle with weight issues?

We may think we burn calories only by exercising, but the truth is we burn calories 24 hours a day, every day. Our bodies are constantly "on" like an engine that's always running. It takes energy for the body to do everything, even things we don't need to think about. It takes energy to breathe, for the heart to beat, for food to digest, for our brains to think. We burn calories even when we sleep.

The minimum number of calories needed to keep the body functioning even if a person were to lie in bed all day doing nothing is called the Basal Metabolic Rate, or BMR. Any activity that increases the BMR beyond basic bodily functions requires extra calories. These activities include talking, walking, playing, laughing, running, dancing, and swimming, just to name a few. So taking into account the BMR, and the activities that your children engage in, how do you know how many calories they are supposed to eat? How does this compare to the amount of calories adults are supposed to eat?

Children, unlike adults, are actively growing. They need calories to build tissues, bones, and muscle. Children are supposed to grow and get bigger, but even during this growing phase they can eat excess calories, and excess calories are stored as extra body fat. The key to a healthy weight for both children and adults is to maintain a balance between the calories eaten and the calories burned.

Table 2.1 shows the number of recommended calories needed at different ages, gender, and activity levels. Study the numbers until you are familiar with the recommendations. Remember, we need calories to sustain us, but any extra calories we eat will be stored as fat, and too much stored fat can be bad for our health. It is good to have a general idea of how many calories you and your child should be eating. You will be amazed to see how many calories are consumed by you in a day, compared to how many calories the body actually needs.

Understanding Basic Nutrition

Carbohydrates

Carbohydrates come from starchy foods and grains such as oat, wheat, barley, and corn. They are in bread, pasta, cereal, some fruits and vegetables, dairy products, and nuts. They can be found in almost every food except for meat products. Carbohydrates provide most of the energy we need in our daily lives. Carbohydrates can be either *simple* or *whole grain*, but in both cases, they are broken down in the body into an even sim-

TABLE 2.1

Daily Calorie (Energy) Recommended for Adults and Children

Children	Sedentary	Active
2–3 years	1,000	1,400
Females	**Sedentary**	**Active**
4–8 years	1,200	1,800
9–13	1,600	2,200
14–18	1,800	2,400
19–30	2,000	2,200
31–50	1,800	2,200
51+	1,800	2,200
Males	**Sedentary**	**Active**
4–8 years	1,400	2,000
9–13	1,800	2,600
14–18	2,200	3,200
19–30	2,400	3,000
31–50	2,200	3,000
51+	2,000	2,800

pler sugar called glucose. The body uses glucose to give cells energy. We believe both adults and children should receive 40–50% of their daily total calories from carbohydrates.

Simple sugars are digested very quickly. Examples of simple sugars that you may find in the list of ingredients on a food label are sucrose (cane or beet sugar), high fructose corn syrup (common in juice drinks), and lactose (sugar found in dairy products).

Examples of products made with simple sugars are juices, ice cream, cookies, and candy. You should try to limit simple sugars in your child's diet as much as possible. They are rapidly absorbed by the body and can raise blood sugar levels. We will discuss why this is important when we talk about diabetes.

Although simple sugars taste sweeter, most children will eat fresh fruits and vegetables if given the opportunity. The reason children may choose sweets over fruit and vegetables is because that's all they have been offered. Try to limit sweets, juice, and soda pop to no more than eight ounces a day, and junk food to no more than 2–3 times a week. Also, replacing refined carbohydrates with whole grains is a good first start. Making these investments in your child's health early in life will pay off later.

Refined Carbohydrates are starchy products that have been stripped of their fiber, vitamins, and minerals. For example, white flour is made from wheat that has been stripped of most of the fiber and other nutrients. Fiber feels rough and removing it makes the flour smoother. Many breads, pasta, and cereals are made from these refined carbohydrates. You can quickly spot refined carbohydrates on the ingredients list. If the list says "enriched flour," that means the fiber, vitamins, and minerals were destroyed during the processing, and then were added back to the finished product.

Whole Grains: Some complex carbohydrates, like wheat, oat or barley contain the whole seed of a grain. These are termed "whole grains." Whole grains have very thick outer shells. This outer shell contains a lot of fiber. Flour made from the whole seed is not digested as quickly as flour made from just the inner part of the seed. Whole grains are an important part of a balanced diet for everyone, including children. When you are shopping for breads, cereals, pasta, or any other "starchy" products, look for ingredients like "whole wheat flour" or "made from whole grains" on the package labels.

Protein

Children need protein to help them grow, build, and maintain strong muscles. Protein is found mainly in meats, dairy products, nuts, and beans. Protein is made up of individual units called amino acids. There are twenty-two amino acids that the body needs to make muscle and other tissues. The body can make thirteen of the twenty-two amino acids, but you have to eat the other nine. These nine are called "essential amino acids." Essential amino acids come from meats, dairy products, nuts, or beans. At least 20–30% of your diet and your child's diet should come from protein. If your child eats a variety of protein from different sources, he or she will get all the essential amino acids. But there is a caution: although diets high in protein are popular as a weight loss strategy, you should avoid these diets for children. There are rare instances when too much protein can be a problem, as in cases of individuals with kidney disease.

Fats

All bodies need some fat. Fat helps to keep us warm, provides cushioning and insulation for our internal organs, and helps to keep our skin soft. Very young children need fat for proper brain development. Of fats, carbohydrates, and protein, fats contain the most calories. One gram of fat contains nine calories compared to four calories for each gram of protein or carbohydrate.

This means that pound for pound, fat will give you more calories than carbohydrates or protein. There are different types of fat: saturated, unsaturated (monounsaturated and polyunsaturated), and trans fats or partially hydrogenated fats. For both children and adults, it is recommended that no more than 30% of daily calorie intake come from fat.

Saturated fats come from animal sources—meats and dairy products (like whole milk, cheese, and ice cream), stick margarine, butter, and lard. These fats are easy to spot because they are solid at room temperature. Although small amounts of saturated fats are not harmful, moderate to large amounts have been linked to high cholesterol, heart disease, and cancer. The American Heart Association (AHA) recommends that no more than 10% of daily caloric intake be from saturated fats for both adults and children.

Unsaturated fats are liquid at room temperature. They come mainly from plant sources. There are two types: monounsaturated and polyunsaturated. Monounsaturated fats can be found in nuts, avocadoes, and oils such as olive, peanut, and canola. Polyunsaturated fat can be found in vegetable, corn, and soybean oil, nuts, and some cold water fish like salmon and tuna. Unsaturated fats in small to moderate amounts can possibly lower cholesterol levels and help to protect the heart. There are some important fats that the body cannot make. These are referred to as *essential fatty acids*. Polyunsaturated fats found in fish such as salmon provide the body with essential fatty acids, such as Omega-3.

Partially hydrogenated or **trans fats** are chemically manufactured from unsaturated fats by a process known as hydrogenation. Hydrogenation forces naturally liquid oils to become solid at room temperature. This process modifies the fat to make it similar to saturated fat. In the body, trans fats act similarly to, or perhaps even worse than, saturated fats. Trans fats have been found to increase the risk for high cholesterol and heart disease. Although many companies today have been forced to remove trans fats from ingredients, you should read all labels and avoid foods with these fats. Trans fats are found in everything from potato chips, cookies, crackers, fried foods, and many other pre-packaged products.

Cholesterol

It's not all bad news

Cholesterol is a soft, waxy substance that is a component of all your body's cells. Despite its negative reputation as being bad for you, cholesterol is an important part of a healthy body. Cholesterol is found in animal products like eggs, dairy products, and meats. The body uses cholesterol to form cell membranes, manufacture hormones, and perform other functions. The problem occurs when we have too much cholesterol circulating in our bloodstream. A high level of cholesterol in the blood, or *hypercholesterolemia*, is a major risk factor for heart disease.

Excess amounts of fat in the diet are dangerous because cholesterol and other fats cannot dissolve in the blood. They have to be transported to and from the cells by special carriers called *lipoproteins*. There are several kinds of lipoproteins, but the ones we will focus on are low-density lipoprotein (LDL) and high-density lipoprotein (HDL).

Low-density lipoprotein (LDL) is "bad" cholesterol and high–density lipoprotein (HDL) is "good" cholesterol. Eating large amounts of foods containing saturated fats can raise a person's "bad" cholesterol, so you should limit your child's as well as your own cholesterol intake to less than 300 mg per day. If there is a family history of heart disease or stroke you may want to try to lower the daily cholesterol intake to less than 200 mg per day for you and your child. Unfortunately, high cholesterol is not uncommon in overweight children. This may raise their risk for developing heart disease at an early age.

In summary, you want to choose foods that contain unsaturated fats and avoid foods with saturated or trans fats. Good sources of fat are nuts, avocadoes, olives, tuna, and salmon. If you must use oil, olive or canola oils are better choices than other vegetable and nut-based oils (like corn, sunflower, or soybean). Children over age two should not eat excessive amounts of saturated fats. Try skim milk instead of whole milk, and limit the amount of junk food like potato chips.

Establishing these habits in young children will help them continue healthy habits into adulthood. While heart attacks are rare in children, we know changes which can eventually lead to a heart attack may start in childhood. Remember, all fats are high in calories and too many calories can cause excessive weight gain, so even good fats should be eaten in small amounts.

Trimming the Fat

Trimming the fat from your diet can start with your choice of meats. Choose lean cuts of meat because they have less fat. Most supermarkets offer a variety of cuts of meat. Leaner cuts of meats are usually more expensive than full-fat cuts, but if you buy larger packages, the prices are often lower. If you can afford to buy a leaner cut of meat, that will save some work in the kitchen later.

If you must buy fattier meats here are some tips to reduce the fat content: First, remove any skin. Skin has a much higher fat content than the actual meat. Prepare the meat with minimum amount of oil. This usually means baking, boiling, or broiling and avoiding pan frying. Some meats can be pan-cooked without oils. (You can use non-stick cooking spray.) There are also oven fry methods using products like Shake N" Bake®. These products are available at the grocery store and can give baked meats a crispy fried–like coating.

You can also cut the fat in your choice of dairy products. Choose lower fat versions of milk, ice cream, and cheese. Try 2% or skim milk instead of whole milk. Try cheese made with 2% milk instead of whole milk. These products may only be slightly more expensive than the full-fat version. Nuts and avocadoes naturally contain a lot of fat. Although they contain good fats, you want to avoid too many calories. These foods should be eaten in moderation. Beans and legumes are a good source of protein and fiber. They are not very expensive and give a sensation of fullness.

Fiber

Fiber is an important component of carbohydrates. It comes in two forms: soluble and insoluble. Soluble fiber is digestible by the body. It acts much in the same way a sponge absorbs water. As it absorbs water in the intestines and mixes with food, it creates a gel-like substance that helps to control how quickly food is digested. Insoluble fiber passes through your stomach and small intestines mostly undigested, but absorbs lots of water in the large intestines, which adds bulk to soften the stools to keep them moving along regularly. The more fiber a food contains, the better the food is for the body. High fiber foods have many benefits, including lowering the incidence of heart disease, decreasing the risk of certain cancers, and maintaining regular bowel movements, among others.

Examples of fiber-rich foods are dark green vegetables, fruit, (fiber is removed in most juice products, even those made from 100% juice), bran cereals, potatoes (both white and sweet), and products made from whole grains like whole wheat flour. It is good for people to eat as much fiber as they can. It is recommended that teenagers and adults get 25–30 grams of fiber a day and younger children (2 -12), get 20 -30 grams a day.

Other Food Additives
Salt

Salt (also known as sodium) makes food taste better and is often used as a preservative. Many people sprinkle salt on their food even when they are eating foods that have already been cooked with salt to further enhance the flavor. Salt is everywhere. Even if you do not use table salt, you may still be consuming a lot of sodium. Did you know a lot of processed meats like luncheon, breakfast, and precooked meats have a lot of salt already added? Even sauces like barbecue sauce, ketchup, and marinades have a lot of salt. Did you know that canned vegetables have a lot of added salt? Frozen vegetables are better then canned vegetables because they usually do not have added salt, provided you buy the plain variety and not those that come with sauces or added flavorings.

Many African Americans suffer from high blood pressure, which can be made worse by consuming a lot of salt. And more and more children and young adults are developing high blood pressure. Limiting salt can help manage high blood pressure. People without high blood pressure should limit salt to no more than 2,400 mg, or one teaspoon per day. While this is the upper limit, you should aim for the lowest amount possible for both yourself and your child, especially if your child is at risk for high blood pressure.

Vitamins and Minerals (including calcium)

Vitamins and minerals help the body to function at its best. They are little helpers for reactions in the body. Vitamins are naturally found in fruits, vegetables, meats, dairy products, and other foods that we eat daily. The lack of vitamins can cause a problem, but vitamin deficiency is very rare in the United States. Despite this, many parents are concerned that their child may not be getting enough vitamins, especially if the child is a picky eater. Usually though, only children with certain medical conditions or those on a lower calorie diet will need extra vitamins. Although vitamin pills will not harm your child if given in the recommended amounts, there are instances when too much of some vitamins, like Vitamin A, can cause problems. Before giving your child added vitamins, consult your pediatrician. Since most children do not need vitamins, this may save you money in the long run. See Table 2.2 for the function and sources of different vitamins and calcium in the body.

TABLE 2.2

Vitamins Function in the Body

Vitamin	Function	Good Source
A	Helps with good eyesight	Carrots, sweet potatoes
C	Maintains healthy bones, teeth, and gums	Fresh or frozen citrus fruits (like oranges) and green vegetables (like broccoli)
D	Helps build strong bones and teeth	Dairy products like milk
E	Antioxidant (help prevent cell damage)	Vegetable oils and whole grains
K	Helps blood to clot when needed	Green, leafy vegetables, milk
Calcium	Important for strong bones and teeth	Dairy products
B vitamins (B_1, B_2, B_3, B_6, B_{12}) folate, biotin and pantothenic acid	Help cells carry out functions	Meat, beans, nuts

Source: "Dietary Guideline for Americans" http://www.health.gov/dietaryguidelines/dga2005/document/html/appendixB.htm

Minerals

Minerals are also little helpers for the body. Calcium is the most important mineral for strong bones and teeth. Children need calcium for proper growth, especially during adolescence when they are growing rapidly. Many food products add calcium as a benefit. All vitamins and minerals are reported as percentages of the recommended daily allowance (RDA) in one serving of the food, in grams or milligrams. You can find vitamins and minerals on just about every food label.

Breaking Down the Nutrition Label

The label on the front of the package may tell you that the food inside is "New and Improved," but it is the label on the back where the real story is told. Food manufacturers are required by law to list the ingredients and the nutritional content of packaged foods on the nutrition label. This is the label that can usually be found on the back or the side of the package. It lists the calories, fat, carbohydrates, and protein contained in one serving of the food. The nutrition label also lists the salt (sodium), sugar, cholesterol, vitamin, and mineral content. It tells you how many grams or milligrams of each it contains, and the percent daily value. The percent daily value, written as "%DV" on the food label, is the percentage of nutrients supplied in one serving of the food if you were aiming to eat 2,000 calories a day. Since children have lower caloric needs, the percent daily value may not be accurate for your child. Also, don't be fooled by the food label! All the information listed is for only *one* serving, while one can or package may actually contain several servings.

The food manufacturers of each product determine the size of the serving, so you need to pay attention to the numbers on the nutrition label.

Serving Size—There may be more than meets the eye

Let us examine a typical food label; let us say it is for a can of beans as shown in Figure 5. It has listed 250 calories per serving. Does the entire can contain one serving? If you answered "true," you would be incorrect. Many people mistakenly think the calories listed on a nutrition label represent the calories for the *entire* package of food. It would seem more sensible to list the calories for the entire package, but that is not how it is done. This can of beans actually contains two servings. (Look at the top section of the label: Servings per Container = 2.) So if you eat the entire can of beans, the total number of calories you will consume is actually 500 (250 calories per serving x 2).

FIGURE 5

Food Label Illustration

Nutrition Facts

Serving Size 1 cup (228g)
Servings Per Container 2

Start Here

Amount Per Serving

Calories 250   Calories from Fat 110

Check calories

% Daily Value*

Total Fat 12g	18%
Saturated Fat 3g	15%
Trans Fat 3g	
Cholesterol 30mg	10%
Sodium 470mg	20%
Potassium 700mg	20%
Total Carbohydrate 31g	10%
Dietary Fiber 0g	0%
Sugars 5g	
Protein 5g	
Vitamin A	4%
Vitamin C	2%
Calcium	20%
Iron	4%

Limit
these

Quick guide
to % DV
5% or less is low
20% or more is high

Get
enough
of these

* Percent Daily Values are based on a 2,000 calorie diet.
Your Daily Values may be higher or lower depending on
your calorie needs.

Footnote

	Calories	2,000	2,500
Total Fat	Less than	65g	80g
Sat Fat	Less than	20g 25g	
Cholesterol	Less than	300mg	300mg
Sodium	Less than	2,400mg	2,400mg
Total Carbohydrate		300g	375g
Dietary Fiber		25g	30g

Source: http://www.cfsan.fda.gov/~dms/label-dl.html

Nutrition in a Nutshell

We've covered a lot here, and you may need to read it more than once to remember it all. But understanding basic facts about carbohydrates, protein, fats, vitamins, and minerals will make it easier to make healthier selections for you and your family. Let us recap the important points:

1. A calorie is a measurement of a unit of energy. Calories in food come from fats, carbohydrates, and proteins. People need different amounts of calories for energy based on their age, gender, and activity level.

2. Eating too many calories and not exercising enough can cause a person to gain weight while eating too few calories can cause a person to lose weight. If you eat the same amount of calories that you use up, your weight will stay the same.

3. A balanced diet for all Americans older than two years of age should have less than 30% of calories from fat, 40–50% of calories from carbohydrates, and 20–30% of calories from protein, with limited cholesterol, salt, and sugar.

4. Carbohydrates can be simple sugars or whole grains. Simple sugars are found in most juices and snacks and should be limited. Refined carbohydrates are found in white starchy products like bread, pasta, and cereal and should be limited.

5. Whole grains are better than simple sugars and refined carbohydrates. Whole grains keep blood sugar more stable than simple sugars or refined carbohydrates.

6. Saturated and trans fat are the worse kind of fats; they can lead to high cholesterol and heart disease. They should be avoided as much as possible. They are found in meats, stick margarine and butter, lard, and some junk foods like potato chips.

7. Polyunsaturated and monounsaturated fats are the best type of fats. They can help lower cholesterol. They are found in things like nuts, vegetable-based oils, avocadoes, and salmon. You should limit your cholesterol intake to less than 300 mg a day.

8. Protein comes mainly from meat, dairy products, nuts, and beans.

9. Lean protein is better then full-fat protein. Try to purchase lean meats, or remove skin and fat from fattier cuts of meat. Try to purchase low fat dairy products like skim milk.

10. Most children do not need extra vitamins. These are already supplied in their diet.

CHAPTER 2 • EXERCISE

Taking Stock – What's in Your Kitchen?

Now that you have learned a lot about nutrition, let's take an inventory of food items in the kitchen and see how you measure up. Now is the time to take stock and make changes if you need to.

Fats and Proteins

Take a peek in the freezer, refrigerator, and pantry. Let's grab some meats like pork bacon, chicken, fish, and beef. Some of these may or may not have a food label. If it has a food label, look at the fat (including saturated fat), carbohydrate, and protein content. Now look at the meat itself. Is there skin? Do you see visible fat? If so, remove the fat before cooking.

Next, look at the nutrition labels for a variety of dairy products (cheeses, milk, and ice creams or yogurt). Turn to the back of the packages and look at the fat content found on the food label. Are you surprised by what you read?

Carbohydrates

Count the number of sweet snacks in your home. Next, select a juice or soda container and look at the ingredients list. What is the first ingredient? What is the second ingredient? Does high fructose corn syrup appear? Now look at the nutrition label on the same bottle. How many grams of sugar does it contain *per serving*? How many grams of fiber? How much does your child drink of this a day? Given what you've learned, are the amounts healthy for your child? Lastly, let us look at bread. First look at the ingredients listed. Does whole or enriched flour appear? (Remember, enriched means refined which is less healthy.) How much fiber is in each serving? Is this mainly a refined carbohydrate or a whole grain?

Let's look in the pantry now. Select a can of vegetables and a sauce. Look at the sodium content, vitamins, and calcium on the nutrition label. Are you surprised at the amount of sodium listed on the package? Are the foods you've selected good sources of vitamins and calcium? Check the beans for fiber content too. Does it fall within the recommended guidelines?

The Healthy Health Detective: Making it Fun

We have added the following worksheet for you to fill in the nutritional value for the foods you normally eat. Make copies of the blank worksheet so that you can do this exercise over and over again. Make reading food labels a game and invite your children to play it with you. Doing this exercise together will let them see how much and what type of nutrients are in their favorite foods. This way you can teach them about healthy eating without preaching. Children love to feel that they have some control over their lives. This is one way to make them feel important, and you are giving them tools they will be able to use for their entire lifetimes.

For this exercise, you will need to select items which have nutrition labels on them. Select one starch, vegetable or fruit (can or frozen), some meat (fresh or frozen), a dairy product, and a bottle of soda or juice. Based on the nutrition labels, which foods are the healthiest? Which are the least healthy?

How did the calories, fat, sugars, and sodium stack up in the foods you have in your home? Are they too high? How can we make better choices? Let us look to the next chapter for solutions in helping you clean up your pantry.

The Healthy Health Detective Kitchen Assessment Table

	Starch	Vegetables or Fruit	Meat	Dairy Product	Soda or juice
Number of servings per package					
Calories					
Fat grams					
Saturated fat grams					
Trans fat grams					
Carbohydrates in grams					
Sugar in grams					
Protein in grams					
Sodium in mg					
% Calcium					
Any vitamins listed?					
Is this food healthy or unhealthy?					

CHAPTER THREE

Can Tasty and Healthy Live Together?

Objectives

- Examine current eating habits in the United States
- Understand proper portion sizes
- Examine healthy choices in your kitchen and the grocery store
- Learn how to prepare healthy meals at home
- Explain the connection between fast food and obesity

So far we have discussed the importance of proper nutrition and maintaining healthy weight in children. You now know how to determine your child's BMI and how to read nutrition labels on food. You also understand how fats, carbohydrates, and protein affect the body. How do we use all we've learned to make good choices in the real world? While making changes at home will help, it only solves one half of the problem. Most families are often on the go; and there are road blocks that make it hard to eat healthy as well. Barriers such as money, dining out, and even cultural norms can have an effect on how and what we eat.

We are as a nation very busy, especially with most parents working outside the home. We don't have time to prepare our own meals, so we eat a lot of fast food, often on the go. We eat everywhere; at home, in the car, at the mall, even at the movies. There is almost no place where we don't have access to food. Food is the guest of honor or the centerpiece at most events. We are expected to eat at most major celebrations: birthdays, retirement parties, graduations, weddings, housewarmings, and bridal and baby showers. Even at funerals, food provides comfort to the mourners. You may be thinking there is nothing wrong with having food at celebrations, and you are absolutely right. But think about how many of these celebrations we have on a monthly basis. How many activities do you and your child attend regularly?

Some people may experience the opposite of this problem. They do not have a lot of money nor do they attend many parties, yet are still overweight. Some people, especially those with limited budgets, may feel food is not always available when they want it. Some people are afraid they may run out of food or not have enough to eat. They may have had this problem in the past or may be currently unemployed, homeless, or are on a fixed budget. Parents may remember when they were young and did not have enough food. They do not want their children to go through the same thing. If you and your family do not have enough to eat or you fear you won't have enough to eat at some point, you may have what psychologists refer to as *food insecurities*. This fear may cause them to eat a lot when given the opportunity. It's no surprise minorities may experience this more than the general population. We can remember growing up and hearing our mothers say, "Eat all of your food because children are starving in Africa." While this might have been true, we always had access to food. Our mothers remembered a time when *they* did not have enough food. It was a blessing to be able to provide for us and they gave us generous portions to let us know how much they cared.

Using food as a token of love is common in many communities. Some parents express love through cooking or giving their family large meals. It's a great thing to show your family you love them, but remember to try to keep it healthy with good, nutritious food. You want everyone to live a long and healthy life.

Portion Sizes

It's no surprise that Americans are among the biggest people on the planet. Few other places on earth have as many overweight people as the United States. We like everything big in America— big cars, big buildings, big houses, and big meals. Think about it, we all like a bargain and many of us think that "bigger is better," but is that really the case for food? Compared to thirty or forty years ago, Americans eat a lot more food today. Do you know the size of a soda bottle has more than doubled from thirty years ago? Thirty years ago the standard size used to be eight ounces; now 20–ounce sodas rule the vending machines. Portion sizes are also getting bigger. The amount of food we eat at one sitting is referred to as *portion size*. On average, portion sizes for products like potato chips, popcorn, hamburgers, and French fries have increased by 40% compared to thirty years ago. Long gone are the days of a hamburger weighing less than a quarter of a pound; today we have "mega burgers," with one-third to a half pound of meat!

Have you also noticed that food servings in restaurants and coffee shops have gotten a lot bigger since you were a kid? The United States Department of Agriculture (USDA) recommends smaller serving sizes than the portion sizes manufacturers and restaurants offer. It's not just what we put on our plates, but also what other people put on our plates that matters. Did you know that an average cookie is 700% larger than the recommended cookie size? Or that in a restaurant, a single serving of pasta can contain your recommended serving for carbohydrates and fat for the entire day? Look at Figure 6. Does it look familiar? Figure 6 shows the serving size of today. Compare the calories we are consuming today with twenty years ago. What a difference! Recommended serving sizes have not changed much, but our portion sizes have gotten much bigger.

Table 3.1 lists the recommended serving size for each of the basic food groups (grains, fruits and vegetables, protein, and dairy products).

The "New" Food Pyramid: Your Guide to Healthy Eating

The United States Department of Agriculture (USDA) redesigned the food pyramid in April 2005 so that it can be customized for people of all ages and activity levels. You can find the new food Pyramid at *www.usda.gov*.

The USDA and the United States Department of Health and Human Services (HHS) make recommendations on the number of calories and number of servings of grains, fruit and vegetables, dairy products, and meats for people of different ages, genders, and activity levels. You can find the recommended number of servings for people older than two years of age on the

FIGURE 6

Comparison of Typical Portion Sizes
Now and Then

	20 Years ago	**Today**
Spaghetti dinner	• 500 calories	• 1,025 calories
	• 1 cup spaghetti with sauce and 3 small meatballs	• 2 cups of pasta with sauce and 3 large meatballs
Soda	• 85 calories	• 250 calories
	• 6.5 ounces of soda	• 20 ounces of soda
Muffin	• 210 calories	• 500 calories
	• 1.5 ounces	• 4 ounces

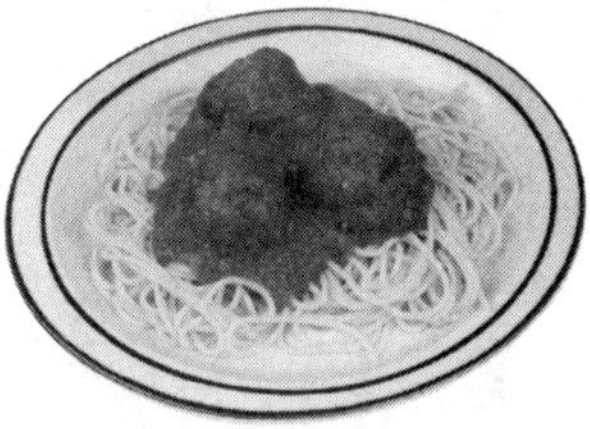

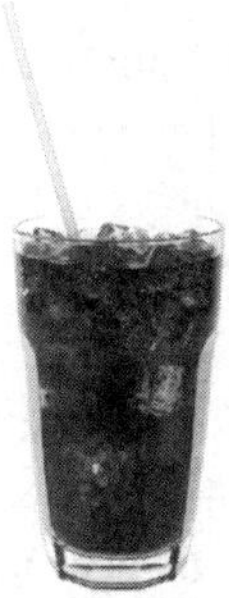

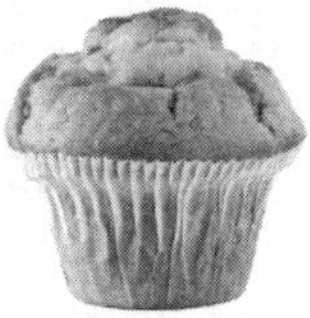

Source: http://hp2010.nhlbihin.net/portion/keep.htm. Last assessed November 30, 2007.

TABLE 3.1

Examples of Recommended Serving Sizes of Food Groups for Older Children and Adults

Food Group	Serving Size	Quick Reminders
Bread, Cereal, Rice, and Pasta	• 1 slice of bread • 1 ounce of ready-to-eat cereal • $\frac{1}{2}$ cup of cooked cereal, rice, or pasta	• $\frac{1}{2}$ cup of grains is about the size of a tennis ball
Fruit	• 1 medium apple, banana, or orange • $\frac{1}{2}$ cup of chopped, cooked, or canned fruit • $\frac{3}{4}$ cup of fruit juice	
Vegetable	• 1 cup of raw leafy vegetables • $\frac{1}{2}$ cup of other vegetables, cooked or chopped, raw • $\frac{3}{4}$ cup of vegetable juice	
Milk, Yogurt, and Cheese	• 1 cup of milk or yogurt • 1 1/2 ounces of natural cheese • 2 ounces of processed cheese	• $1\frac{1}{2}$ ounces of cheese is equivalent to a pair of dice
Meat, Poultry, Fish, Dry Beans, Eggs, and Nuts	• 2–3 ounces of cooked lean meat, poultry, or fish • $\frac{1}{2}$ cup of cooked dry beans • 1 egg counts as 1 ounce of lean meat • 2 tablespoons of peanut butter or $\frac{1}{3}$ cup of nuts count as 1 ounce of meat	• 3 ounces of meat is about the size of a deck of cards

1 cup = 8 ounces (OZ.)

For children aged one through six, use the "one tablespoon of food per year of life" as a serving size. Example, if a child is four, then he or she should receive 4 tablespoons of vegetables, carbohydrates and meats.

Source: Department of Health and Human Services and U.S. Department of Agriculture. Dietary Guidelines for Americans, 2005. 6th Edition, Washington, DC: U.S. Government Printing Office, January 2005

Internet at *www.mypyramid.gov*. The guidelines on this Web site replace the old "one-size-fits-all" food pyramid. You can also find a customized food plan for an active 5–year old on this site, which is user-friendly and contains interactive tools for children and parents. (If you do not have a computer at home, most public libraries have computers that can be used for free.)

Now that we have discussed the importance of understanding the difference between the amount of food one should consume versus the amount of food we actually consume daily, let's apply our knowledge to everyday life.

Making Over Your Kitchen for a Healthier Environment

For some families, the idea of buying more expensive cuts of meat to cut down on the amount of fat they consume is simply not an option. And the cost of food is increasing everyday. If you think your family cannot afford enough groceries, check with your state agencies. The Special Supplemental Nutrition Program for Women, Infants and Children (WIC) assists women with children less than five years of age who cannot afford nutritious foods. The eligibility requirements to join WIC differ from state to state. You should contact your local department of health for more information about the program.

You may also want to visit several different grocery stores and compare prices for products you buy on a regular basis. Make sure to clip coupons as well. You can find hundreds of dollars worth of coupons in the weekend edition of most newspapers. These papers usually cost one to two dollars. Also make sure you get items on sale. Sale items change weekly, so if you see something good, stock up on it. If you are on a budget, buying cheaper foods will allow you to stretch your food-buying dollars, but as dis-cussed cheaper foods are often loaded with more fat, salt, and sugar. Thus you should be aware when you are making a purchase.

If none of the above suggestions help and it comes down to a healthier version of a food which is more expensive than the less healthy version, ask yourself these questions?

1. Is the price cheaper if I buy in bulk?

    • Sometimes the more you buy, the cheaper the price per pound or per package. If you know your family will eat a lot of a particular food, it may be worth the invest-ment to buy more and stock up.

2. Does the less expensive version contain more fat?

    • This may be more common for some beef and pork products. Cheaper cuts of beef and pork usually contain more fat than leaner cuts of meat.

3. Is there a product in between the most expensive, healthier item and the cheaper, less healthy item?

    • For example, boneless, skinless chicken breasts are very good for you compared to chicken wings, but they are almost always two to three times more expensive. A good compromise is chicken thighs. Although they contain more fat than skinless chicken breast, the skin can easily be removed to eliminate a lot of the fat and they usually cost only slightly more than chicken wings.

If your children accompany you to the grocery store, play the Healthy Health Detective game mentioned in Chapter Two. Let them help you make a list of the foods you would like to purchase *before* getting to the grocery store; this will help you stay focused on your mission. At the store, encourage the kids to read the labels and encourage them to make some of the healthier food choices with you.

You now know that healthier alternatives will have fewer calories, and less fat, sugar or salt. If you have use of a computer, we encourage you to look for lower fat recipes for your favorite foods, or you may want to invest in a low-fat recipe book. You may be surprised to learn that lower fat foods can be quite tasty!

Use Table 3.2 which we created to help you shop for healthier versions of your child's favorite foods.

From the Grocery Store to the Table

Children become more interested in adopting healthy food choices when two basic needs are met. First, children are more likely to eat what they help put on the table. Allow your child to assist in planning meals, making the grocery list, unpacking the groceries, and preparing the meals. Allowing children to participate in preparing meals provides an opportunity to discuss the labels on food packages and to discuss the importance of overall nutrition. This is also an opportunity to compare food products such as white versus whole grain bread or whole milk versus 2% milk, using the food labels to show the differences in calories, carbohydrates, and fat. Comparisons of water and beverages with added sugars can also assist in encouraging kids to choose water over sugary drinks. Children can also assist in selecting healthy

TABLE 3.2

Healthy Grocery Store Choices

Common Kid Food	Healthier Alternative	Why the alternative is healthier
Regular juice and soda pop	• "Light" or no-sugar-added juices • Water	• All soda pop and many juices are simply "sugar water" and have very little nutritional value. The actual fruit is much better for the child than the juice. • Water does not contain calories.
Whole Milk	• Low fat or skim milk	• Low fat and skim milk contain less fat and calories than whole milk. Note: all children under two years of age need whole milk.
Cheese products	• Cheese products made with 2% or fat-free milk	• Contains less fat and calories than regular full-fat cheeses.
White bread (and similar products)	• "Whole wheat" and "multi-grain" bread	• Contain more complex carbohydrates and less refined carbohydrates than white bread. • Contain more complex carbohydrates and less refined carbohydrates than white bread.
Cereal (both cold and warm)	• "Less sugar" or "no sugar added" cereals • "Whole grains"	• Less sugar is always better.

Common Kid Food	Healthier Alternative	Why the alternative is healthier
Meat (beef)	• Turkey if available. Ground turkey instead of ground beef or reduced fat products.	• Beef tends to be a very high calorie, high fat meat. The substitutes contain less fat and calories. Fat on beef products can be reduced by trimming all visible fat. Leaner cuts of beef and reduced-fat beef products tend to be more expensive than regular cuts of beef or products.
Meat (pork)	• Turkey if available (for example, using turkey instead of pork to season vegetables). • Leaner cuts of pork	• Pork tends to contain a lot of salt and so can the substitutes, so watch the salt (sodium) content. In general, turkey products are lower in fat than pork products. Fat on pork products can be reduced by trimming all visible fat.
Meat (poultry, like chicken and turkey)	• White meat • Skinless meat	• A lot of fat is found in the skin. White meat has fewer calories than dark meat.
Fish	• All fish	• Just about all fish is good for you. Fresh and frozen fish will have less salt than canned varieties. Avoid fried fish as it will have more calories than fish that has been broiled or sautéed.

continued on next page

continued from previous page

Common Kid Food	Healthier Alternative	Why the alternative is healthier
Fruits	• Fresh fruits • Frozen fruits • Canned fruit in "light syrup" or no sugar added	• Fresh fruit is the best, then frozen. Canned fruit can have added sugars, so look at the labels to avoid this.
Vegetables	• Fresh vegetables • Frozen vegetables • Canned vegetables, "low salt"	• Fresh vegetables are the best, then frozen. Canned vegetables can have a lot of salt so be careful and try to get the lower-salt versions.
Fats and oils	• Olive oil or vegetable oil; soft margarine or butter; "light" mayonnaise and salad dressings	• Avoid lard and shortening. The fat they contain is particularly bad (saturated and trans fat). • Regular mayonnaise and salad dressings are packed with calories.
Sweets and snacks	• Reduced calorie, reduced sugar, "light" or "no sugar added" snacks • Baked snacks • "Whole grain" snacks • Small bags or mini versions of sweets	• As you already know, most snacks and sweets are "empty" calories, but you can still have them. Just look for ones that are healthier or smaller versions of the real thing.

snacks and stocking the refrigerator with fresh fruit and vegetables. By allowing your child to participate, he or she can begin to take responsibility for his or her health at an earlier age.

Secondly, involving children in meal preparation gives parents another opportunity to serve as positive role models for healthy living. Children have a greater chance of becoming healthy eaters if the behavior is viewed as a family activity led by the heads of the household. Eating as a family allows the parents to model good eating habits to their children and also serves as a time to discuss the role healthy food choices play in how well they perform in school and athletics. After all, parents are children's most important teachers.

Now that you have chosen items from the grocery store, use these tips to prepare healthy, nutritious meals at home:

1. Offer your child three meals and two healthy snacks a day. (This is good for adults too.) Foods such as chips and sweets should be viewed as occasional snacks.
2. Include fresh vegetables at every meal. Try having fresh fruit for desserts. The entire family should aim to eat at least five servings of fruits and vegetables each day.
3. Avoid using high-fat and high-salt products to season vegetables. (For example, try turkey to season vegetables instead of pork.)
4. Bake, broil, or steam meats, poultry, and fish; avoid frying in oil or grease. Try using non-stick cooking oil sprays to reduce the amount of oil when pan frying.
5. Try baking meats with bread crumbs for a crispy, crunchy coating. (Some cuts of meat are pre-prepared in grocery stores.)

6. Limit the amount of sugar and salt you add to food. Try to stick to complex carbohydrates and try to avoid refined carbohydrates as described in Chapter Two.
7. Offer your child their suggested serving size instead of piling the plate with food. If your child wants a second helping, give him or her vegetables first. Use smaller plates to make the plate appear more filled up.
8. If your child does not want to eat all of his or her appropriate portion size, put it in the refrigerator until later. If he or she gets hungry again, offer the same meal.
9. Allow your child to drink water or milk with his or her meals.
10. Find activities to keep your child busy in between meal times.

Dining Out

Eating out doesn't mean overeating. Fast food has slowly taken over our country, homes, and even our cars! On an average day in America, 20–25% of the country eats some type of fast food and almost fifty cents of every dollar spent on food is for food prepared outside the home. That is a lot and that's just for adults. The numbers are even higher for children. Today, 30% of children eat fast food every day compared to only 10% thirty years ago. Why is this so bad? There are several reasons:

- Fast food is loaded with lots of calories, fat, salt, and sugar.
- Children who eat fast food eat fewer fruits and vegetables.

- It is hard to know exactly how many calories you eat when you eat out.
- You have less control and you may not even be aware of what is in the food you're eating.

Many fast food restaurants constantly increase portion sizes, making super sizes the standard sizes. The offerings on a plain cheeseburger have gone from a single patty to two or more patties. A single serving of soft drinks can be as large as a liter. Even breakfast items are getting bigger, piling on more meat, eggs, and cheese. Don't forget most of the food is fried in oil (sometimes lard or trans fat) which significantly increases the calorie and fat content of a food that is usually considered healthy, such as chicken breast.

We all know that most fast foods are high in calories and low in nutrients. Thankfully, due to recent consumer pressure, many fast food chains and restaurants have begun to make their nutrition information public. You can also check online at the company's Web site for nutrition information and calorie content of your favorite fast foods.

You may not be able to eliminate fast food from your child's diet altogether, but you can make healthier choices from fast food menus. Here are some quick tips for selecting healthier foods when dining out:

1. Encourage children younger than ten to order food from the children's menu.
2. Encourage them to choose fruit or yogurt as a side instead of pie or cookies.

3. Choose vegetables and salads. (Watch the amount of dressing.)
4. Look for items or meals with less than 500 calories. Some restaurant chains highlight these items.
5. Limit the amount of soda or juice to 8 ounces and encourage your child to drink water as well.
6. Limit the amount of fried foods.
7. If the portion size is too big for your child, wrap half of it up and take it home for another meal. If your child does not want the entire meal, it's okay to throw it away. You may feel like you are wasting money, but you are saving your child many calories by not forcing him or her to eat all of it. Next time, consider ordering less food.
8. Order small, plain desserts if your child must have dessert.
9. Remember you are in control at restaurants; help your child make healthy choices.
10. Eat slowly.

We don't want to scare you into thinking that your child can never eat any "fun" foods, but it should be done in moderation. As a parent, you have to weigh all of your options when making food choices for the family. Here are some tips to remember.

1. Remember portion sizes. We eat larger portions today then we did thirty years ago. You determine what the proper size should be for your child, not the food manufacturers or the restaurants.
2. Eat three meals and two snacks a day.

3. Plan your trips to the grocery store. Look for healthy alternatives to common foods that kids eat.
4. Stock your kitchen with healthy choices.
5. Offer fruit and vegetables at every meal, preferably five servings a day. Offer lean meats that are baked, broiled, or boiled.
6. Try to make mealtime "family time" as much as possible. Try to find activities for your child in between mealtimes.
7. Never force your child to eat. Children are very good at eating what their bodies need. If your child is under medical supervision, check with your child's doctor first.
8. Limit visits to fast foods and restaurants as much as possible. If you go to fast food restaurants, make healthier choices.
9. Get to know the nutritional information for items on the menus in your favorite fast food restaurants.
10. Limit juice, soda pop, and snacks; remember, moderation is the key.

CHAPTER 3 • EXERCISE

Encourage your child to participate in this exercise with you.

1. Determine your child's daily calorie needs by using Table 2.1 on page 24 and enter the information in the box.

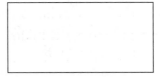

2. If you have access to a computer, go to *www.mypyramid.gov* and print out your child's individualized food plan.

3. Based on the information in this chapter, write out your grocery list for a week. Once in the grocery store, compare the prices of some of the healthier foods to the regular versions.

4. Think about one restaurant you and your child like to visit. Go to their Web site and look up the nutrition information of some of your favorite foods. Look at small sizes versus larger sizes. If you do not have access to a computer, go to the restaurant and ask for its nutrition information guide.

A B C's of Eating Disorders
Anorexia Nervosa, Bulimia, and Compulsive Eating

Objectives

- Become familiar with common eating disorders such as anorexia, bulimia, and compulsive eating
- Understand the incidence of common eating disorders within different communities
- Recognize the warning signs of an eating disorder
- Understand the effects of overweight on self-esteem

We have discussed with you the importance of living a healthy lifestyle and how to maintain a healthy lifestyle. We have covered the dangers of excess weight and how excess weight may impact your children. However, we must be clear that children should not be pushed too hard so as to make them become obsessed with their weight and appearance, as the pressure can have many bad effects—both physical and mental. The same is true for adults. If you have continued feelings of concern about your child's weight, you should seek professional help. Discuss your concerns with a healthcare professional. While the ultimate goal is to make sure your child is healthy, he or she may be dealing with other issues beyond your immediate control. His or her issues can result in developing an eating disorder.

In general, an eating disorder develops when a person becomes extremely obsessed with what they eat and how they look. People with eating disorders become preoccupied with their weight and usually have a misperception of their weight. They are so afraid of gaining weight, they do things that are very unhealthy and can be life threatening. Although the obsession is with physical appearance, eating disorders can stem from psychological problems like depression. People suffering from eating disorders may not want to eat at all; they may starve themselves and become underweight as in *anorexia nervosa* (AN). Some people may eat small amounts most of the time, but then go on binges, eating very large amounts at one sitting. This is known as binge eating. After binge eating or even after normal eating, some people vomit up their food to avoid gaining weight (purging). People who binge then purge suffer from *bulimia*.

Who is at risk?

When you imagine someone with an eating disorder, what do they look like? Do they look like you? As you read this, you may be thinking "these things don't happen in my community or family." The truth is anyone can develop an eating disorder, regardless of gender or ethnic group, and, to some extent, age. According to the National Association of Anorexia Nervosa and Associated Disorders, seven million women and one million men in the U.S. suffer from some type of eating disorder. Historically there has been more pressure on women to look good than on men. Women sometimes wear makeup, style their hair, and have a lot of clothes to make their appearance more attractive for themselves and their mates. As trends change, sometimes thin is in. At other times, rounder figures may be popular. Some women try to change themselves to fit with the trend. One can say that this may be true for men, but to a lesser extent. Men usually fulfill their role in society by being the breadwinner, so they usually concentrate more on building wealth than adapting to what is considered attractive. Given this history, it is not surprising that women would be more concerned about their appearance and weight than men.

Eating disorders often begin in the teenage years. Early puberty (around eleven) and late puberty (around seventeen) appear to be heavily hit ages. Each age marks a milestone of change for the developing teenager and young adult. At the start of puberty, girls' bodies are changing in preparation for their periods. Fat begins to fill in a once thin frame. This new growth can be difficult for a young girl to handle. Many studies have shown that girls as young as eight and nine years of age have reported behaviors that are consistent with eating disorders. Late puberty marks another period of change. As teenagers enter young adulthood, they become extremely concerned with "ideals" of beauty. It is during this time that young girls may start to feel pressure to look like the usually very thin women on television and in magazines. Also, young girls may be trying to assert control over their lives, which may cause conflict with their parents. Controlling their eating can be a psychological attempt to regain control in the rest of their lives. In a time of confusion between being told what to do by their parents and deciding for themselves what is best, eating appears to the child to be the only feature which he or she can completely control.

If you think that only White girls suffer from this, you may be surprised to know that African-American and Latina girls suffer too. Overall, minority girls do say they are more satisfied with their bodies compared to their White peers, but they also report behaviors like binge eating, vomiting, and taking laxatives (medicine that makes you have a bowel movement) in order to lose or maintain weight. As America becomes more of a melting pot, cultures are becoming more mixed. This means that minorities are becoming more and more a part of and being exposed to mainstream culture. This means that some of them are feeling pressures to also be very thin. Even in hip-hop culture, which is more often seen as the culture of inner city youth, women in front of the camera in that industry are often thin and show their bodies. Some young girls may want to imitate them and become willing to do whatever it takes to achieve a thinner look.

In summary, although eating disorders are not as common in minority communities as in White communities, they do occur. Mental, social, psychological, genetic, or environmental factors can contribute to the development of an eating disorder. We encourage parents to be aware of the signs and behavorial differences in their child. Let's take a look at some of the most common disorders.

What Is Anorexia Nervosa?

Anorexia nervosa occurs when a person is so afraid of being fat or gaining weight that he or she restricts his or her eating almost to the point of starvation. It often occurs in young women and teens. Teenagers and children with anorexia nervosa may be perfectionists who seek approval from friends and family and often severely underweight. Regardless of how thin they become, a person with anorexia nervosa considers himself or herself to be overweight. Not only do they restrict eating to the extreme, they spend the majority of their time thinking of ways to control their weight. They may eat extremely slowly while thinking about each bite. Many normal daily activities are replaced with thoughts of food and weight loss. There is constant thought about the number of fat grams in foods and calorie intake. Some people with anorexia exercise beyond what is reasonable. Sometimes a person with anorexia can diet and exercise to the point of death. An example of an anorexia nervosa patient may be a sixteen year-old female who is 5' 2" tall but only weighs 90 pounds. Her calculated BMI (90 / 62 / 62 x 703) is 16.5! This is definitely underweight (when referring to the chart). Despite her extreme thinness, when looking in the mirror she sees herself as overweight. This distorted image and overwhelming desire to be thin begins the downward cycle of dieting, extreme exercise, diet pills, and laxatives used to desperately try to lose weight.

The Physical Effects of Anorexia Nervosa

Although there are numerous physical problems with overweight and obesity, the physical effects of anorexia can be just as bad. Most of the physical problems in anorexia are due to poor nutrition. Anorexia may cause malnutrition and dehydration. Malnutrition occurs because the body is not getting enough vitamins, minerals, and nutrients to keep it healthy. Malnutrition affects the body much the same way running the engine without gasoline affects a car. Without gasoline, a car will eventually stall and leave its passengers short of their destination. Anorexia nervosa can lead to stunted growth, profound weakness, loss of body fat and muscle, sensitivity to cold, hair loss, and extra facial or body hair due to a lack of protein in the diet. It can also do weird things, like turning the skin orange. This is caused by a buildup of a pigment called carotene (the same pigment that gives carrots their bright color).

Girls who become anorexic will often stop menstruating due to malnutrition and excessive loss of weight. A particularly difficult problem in anorexia is osteoporosis. Osteoporosis occurs when the thickness and density of the bones decrease and the bones become much lighter. The lighter the bones, the more easily they can break, leading to painful and deforming fractures.

Dehydration can occur when not enough fluid is taken. The body normally contains a great deal of water that needs to be constantly replaced. Without enough water, the body becomes extremely dry and cannot carry out its normal functions. Both malnutrition and dehydration become worse the longer the disorder remains untreated.

There are many signs and symptoms associated with anorexia (see Table 4.1), but they do not all have to be present for a diagnosis to be made.

What is Bulimia?

Like anorexia, bulimia is an illness that usually affects young women in their teen years, but younger children can also be affected.

TABLE 4.1

Signs and Symptoms of Anorexia

Physical Signs of Anorexia	Physical Symptoms of Anorexia
Stunted growth	Heightened sensitivity to cold
Failure of breast development	Constipation
Dry skin	Bloated feeling after eating
Orange hue to skin	Dizziness
Cold hands and feet	Irregular periods
Slow heart rate	Poor sleep
Swelling in the ankles	Early morning wakening
Muscle weakness	Not being able to get pregnant

Source: Info from http://www.mayoclinic.com

As with people with anorexia nervosa, their feelings of self worth are based on their weight and shape. But unlike children with anorexia who starve themselves, children with bulimia experience an uncontrollable urge to eat huge quantities of food known as binging in a short amount of time, and then purge the food. Purging is when food that was recently eaten is intentionally removed by throwing up or taking laxatives. Children and young people who are bulimic may also exercise excessively in an attempt to undo the damage done by binging. They then feel very guilty and unhappy about their behavior. It may be difficult to know if your child is bulimic as the excessive eating is usually done in secret. Children with bulimia may be harder to recognize than children with anorexia because they may have a normal weight or may even be overweight. On the surface those suffering with bulimia may appear "normal," but may have underlying psychological issues. Teenagers with bulimia may participate in more activities that have poor long-term consequences such as early sexual initiation, sexual promiscuity, and experimentation with drugs, alcohol, and tobacco. In one study, one-third of all teenagers with bulimia indicated they smoked tobacco, used marijuana, or drank alcohol at least weekly. Stealing and thoughts about suicide were also more common in individuals with bulimia. Children and teenagers with bulimia often had a history of mood changes, family problems, or sexual abuse.

While bulimia may be more common than anorexia, deaths associated with these illnesses are more common from anorexia.

The Physical Effects of Bulimia

All eating disorders cause physical harm to the body and can lead to lifelong medical problems, including heart, liver, and kidney disease. People with bulimia frequently experience tooth decay and gum disease which comes from vomiting repeatedly. These dental problems are caused by acid in the stomach. Think of battery acid. Most people know that if you get battery acid on your skin it will eat into your skin. When a person with bulimia repeatedly vomits, strong stomach acids come into frequent contact with the teeth. Over time, this can lead to loss of tooth enamel, the coating that protects the teeth. The strong acids also cause damage to the gums. (See the signs and symptoms of Bulimia in Table 4.2).

TABLE 4.2

Signs and Symptoms of Bulimia

Physical Signs of Bulimia	Physical Symptoms of Bulimia
Damaged teeth and gums	Self-induced vomiting
Swollen salivary glands in the cheeks	Inappropriate laxative use
Bloating	Excessive exercise
Sores in the throat and mouth	Constantly using the bathroom following eating
Dehydration	Irregular periods
Dry skin	Can't control eating
Scars and calluses on knuckles or hands	Fatigue

Source: http://www.mayoclinic.com

What is Binge Eating?

Binge eating, otherwise known as compulsive overeating, is strongly linked to obesity. Unlike anorexia and bulimia, it is thought that compulsive overeaters are mainly adults. However, due to the recent increase in the numbers of overweight children, compulsive overeating may be spreading to include children. Binge eaters will eat more than 2,500 calories in one sitting or in less than two hours. In other words, binge eaters may eat more then their total recommended daily allowance in just one meal! This is followed by strong feelings of guilt and unhappiness. These feelings are not as bad as those seen in individuals with bulimia. Unlike bulimia, binge eating is not followed by purging.

Given the often easy access to food for some children, binge eating may be the most common eating disorder in minority communities. Whether it is Sunday dinner, celebrations, or special occasions, if you and your children have access to large amounts of tasty food, it may be difficult to stop even though you have had more than your share. For some people, just seeing food makes them crave it. Think about it. If you put out three hamburgers on a plate instead of one, for some children it may be hard to resist all three mentally even if they are satisfied physically. Some children also sneak and eat food late at night when no one is awake. These behaviors are examples of binge eating.

The Physical Effects of Binge Eating

Binge eating frequently leads down the path to overweight or obesity. In turn, the diseases linked to obesity—heart disease, stroke, high blood pressure, diabetes, high cholesterol, arthritis, asthma, and obstructive sleep apnea—can be seen in people suffering from this type of eating disorder. As in obesity, long-term changes in diet and exercise can undo the physical damage of binge eating.

As seen in Table 4.3, some of the signs of the different eating disorders may overlap. All eating disorders are linked to self-esteem and the person's view of his/her weight and shape. This may be the number one reason why childhood obesity is not just about weight. Lack of self-esteem due to appearance or perceived appearance can lead to more serious illness and disorders, which may lead to death.

TABLE 4.3

Signs and Symptoms of Binge Eating

Physical Signs of Binge Eating	Physical and Emotional Symptoms of Binge Eating
May be normal weight, overweight, or obese	Eating to the point of discomfort
Shortness of breath	Hoarding of food
Excessive sweating	Eating alone
Leg or joint pain	Hiding empty containers
Out of breath after light activity	Depression
Weight gain despite dieting	Sees food as a good friend
	Poor sleeping habits
	Feels that eating is out of control

Source: http://www.mayoclinic.com

TABLE 4.4

Warning Signs of Eating Disorders

	Refusing to Eat	Constant Dieting	Excessive Exercise	Sensitive to Cold	Self-Induced Vomiting After Binging	Irregular Periods	Binge Eating	Constantly Thinking About Food	Laxative, Diet Pills, or Diuretic Abuse
Anorexia	X	X	X	X					
Bulimia			X		X	X	X	X	X
Binge Eating							X	X	

Psychological Issues

The damage caused by eating disorders extends beyond the obvious physical changes. Eating disorders can cause a person to feel badly about himself or herself. Depression, shame, and guilt are common emotions associated with eating disorders.

Problems associated with eating disorders are not confined to the person with the eating disorder. They can also cause pain and suffering to family and friends. Eating disorders can cause family members to blame themselves, leading to feelings of guilt and shame. Family and friends may struggle with feelings of frustration over how to help their loved one as well as understanding how and why the illness occurs. Dealing with eating disorders can be difficult for everyone involved. It can have a harmful effect on the family. Children with eating disorders have a greater chance of having mood swings, which can further threaten their relationships with friends and family members.

Young people who develop eating disorders often begin with dieting. They believe that weight loss will lead them to feeling better about themselves. What happens instead is that under-eating, binge eating, and purging have the exact opposite result. Teens with eating disorders often struggle with feeling out of control. They may also feel guilty about their behavior and may feel that others are watching them and are waiting to confront them about their behavior. Teenagers with eating disorders may adopt compulsive behaviors like refusing to let food touch their lips or cutting food into tiny bite-size pieces. They often feel alone and hopeless and estranged from everyone and everything. Because of changes that take place in the brain due to long-term inadequate nutrition intake, the teenager with binge eating and purging may not make logical choices. Once they begin to recover, it takes time for the brain to readjust both chemically and physically.

Why Do Some Children Have These Issues?

Many factors are needed to produce an eating disorder; a combination of life experiences and environmental/social issues often contribute to the problems that lead to developing eating disorders. When these risk factors are combined with stressful events, including family strife, high expectations, low involvement of parents, and low self-esteem, the result may be the beginning of an eating disorder.

There is a delicate balance between being motivated to get healthy (and lose some extra weight if necessary) and feeling good about yourself. Lower self-esteem has not been linked to being overweight in minority children as much as in Whites, but that may change. Many television shows promote the idea that "thin is in." Many sitcoms make fun of overweight characters. We all have memories of overweight classmates who were teased to tears. We saw the outside effects but were unaware of the long-term consequences. Did those classmates in time lose weight and grow up to be healthy and happy? Did they continue to gain weight but still grow up to be happy adults? Did the abuse caused by name calling or simply being picked last for the neighborhood softball games create lifetime scars? Time has shown that the effects of childhood teasing can indeed be long-term. Negative actions towards overweight children by other kids can create negative and often destructive results. And can cause children to have social problems when they become adults.

Let's look at how overweight children are treated by their peers and the effect it can have on them. As cultures become more and more mixed, we may start to see more of these problems in Black and Hispanic children. We want to make you aware of some of the problems your child may have in an effort to create a dialogue between you and your child.

Unfortunately, anytime children are different they can become victims of abuse both by other children and adults. There are four major types of abuse experienced by overweight children: verbal, relational, physical, and sexual abuse are all possible. As a child's weight increases, the chances of being a victim of abuse increase with every pound. Verbal abuse, perhaps one of the most common types of abuse, is teasing or name calling. Overweight children are frequently the target of cruel jokes and hurtful names. Relational abuse involves losing friends or simply being left out of social activities like slumber parties and pick-up basketball games. Physical abuse, which is less common, involves hitting and pushing. Physical abuse may happen less because overweight children may be seen as a threat due to their larger sizes. Sexual abuse may be linked to the low self-esteem an overweight child may have.

One study found that overweight and obese children and teenagers were more likely to be verbally or physically bullied compared to their average weight peers. Also, girls were more likely to be victims of relational victimization than boys. However, many overweight children respond to teasing and name calling by becoming bullies themselves, especially when they become teenagers. This behavior may begin as early as fifteen years of age. Overweight children can inflict the same types of verbal, physical, and relational abuse on others at this age. It may surprise you to know that boys are more likely to engage in relational and verbal bullying, while girls are more likely to engage in physical bullying. In short, overweight children victimized by their peers frequently progress into teenage bullies themselves.

Long-Term Effects

The long-term psychological effect on children because of their weight is sometimes shocking and can ultimately influence their social and economic success in life. As children grow and develop into teenagers, their sense of well-being is often determined by feeling accepted by their peers. An overweight child can face a lot of embarrassing situations daily. Going to a pool party or just dressing for gym class can be an uncomfortable experience. Overweight children who participate in sports often face shame by being picked last for the team.

Being teased is a constant problem for overweight children. Frequent teasing of overweight children can have poor effects on their self-esteem. While being picked on threatens the self-esteem of all children, overweight kids may be more at risk. Beginning at age ten, overweight girls and boys can show a decrease in self-esteem and their school performance. Overweight children may also begin to feel more loneliness, sadness, tiredness, and nervousness than other children. This may come from social isolation if they are rejected by other kids. The beginning of adolescence appears to be a crucial time when peer acceptance is an important part of a teen's perception of self worth. Isolation and boredom may lead to an increase in risky behavior, such as smoking and alcohol use, which can also have bad effects on long-term health.

Extracurricular Activity

Sports and other extracurricular activities may also play a role in eating disorders. Certain athletes, girls and boys alike, especially wrestlers, gymnasts, and distance runners, whose performance is largely linked to body size are at greater risk for developing eating disorders. Girls who participate in activities such as modeling, ballet, or cheerleading may feel pressured to keep their bodies at a certain weight. Therefore, they may start experimenting with fad diets or quick weight loss solutions which may eventually lead to an eating disorder. Boys involved in sports such as wrestling are more likely to develop an eating disorder because of the emphasis on weight. Wrestlers are often pressured to stay within their weight class. This is known as "making weight." Therefore a 215–pound wrestler who gains ten pounds may binge and purge in an effort to stay within his weight class.

If your child is involved in a sport where body size is important, your child's coach can be an ally in spotting the early signs of an eating disorder. Due to the risk of eating disorders in sports where success is determined by a lower weight, the National Athletic Association encourages involvement of coaches and trainers to become familiar with the signs and symptoms of eating disorders and to refer at-risk athletes for additional care as needed.

Genetics

As it does with many other illnesses, genetics can play a role in the development of eating disorders. Studies have been done with twins to see if genes indeed play a role. These studies show that an eating disorder in the immediate family increases the likelihood of an eating disorder in another family member. The most recent studies suggest that a gene that is responsible for regulating a hormone known as *serotonin* may be responsible. Serotonin is often called the "feel good" hormone because it affects our moods and how we feel. Serotonin also helps control eating; high serotonin levels cause feelings of calmness. While the genes responsible for eating disorders remain unknown, the mixing of genes and environment seem to trigger an eating disorder. Starving the body, for example, is a change in environment that can cause or "turn on," an eating disorder. Although many studies point to different results about the role of genetics on eating disorders, what does remain clear is that genes play a huge role in the development of both bulimia and anorexia.

Diagnosing an eating disorder requires a thorough physical exam, including a weight and height assessment; it also requires the health care provider to ask questions designed to uncover an eating disorder. Going to your pediatrician for regularly scheduled checkups will allow for early detection of a problem. Issues such as drug use, cessation of periods, or problems with teeth can help your doctor in considering the possibility of an eating disorder.

The Doctor's Visit

The questions listed in Table 4.5 are designed to show some of the signs and symptoms of eating disorders. If your child is diagnosed with an eating disorder, you will need to get him or her thoroughly evaluated by specialists to develop an appropriate

TABLE 4.5

Screening Questions to Help Identify an Eating Disorder in Children

Screening Questions

- What is the least you have weighed in the last year?
- What do you think your weight should be?
- How much do you exercise, how often, and how long?
- Is there any binge eating?
- Is there any history of purging?
- Have you ever been treated for an eating disorder?
- Do you have regular periods?
- Do you use cigarettes, alcohol, or any illicit drugs?
- Have you noticed any change in your tolerance to cold temperatures?
- Have you experienced any dizziness lately?
- Have you experienced any bloating after eating?

treatment plan. This should include a nutritionist and psychologist who may reveal the presence of underlying depression and anxiety disorders.

Pay special attention to any of the possible warning signs listed in the following table and bring them to the attention of your child's doctor. Early diagnosis of an eating disorder can mean early intervention. When diagnosed early, the physical and mental problems associated with eating disorders can be reduced.

TABLE 4.6

Eating Disorder Warning Signs

Eating Disorder Warning Signs

- Overly concerned with their body image
- Always going on a diet
- Eating huge amounts of food at a time without stopping
- Embarrassed or guilty about eating
- Describing self as feeling fat
- Sneaking food or lying about what they eat
- Feels bad about self
- Girls no longer have normal periods
- Obsessed with the topic of food
- Using diet pills, laxatives, or diuretics

Source: http://www.mayoclinic.com

What Can You Do As a Parent?

Encourage your children to feel safe and secure about their size and appearance. Work on promoting a healthy body and positive self-esteem based upon internal traits such as honesty, compassion, and integrity. Discuss the importance of respect for self and others as it relates to healthy options for dealing with problems. Watch television, read magazines, and talk about the images that you see. Note what messages are being directed at your children about body image and beauty. Talk with them about what truly matters as far as beauty, with a focus on accepting differences in shapes and sizes. Openly discuss the possible results of peer pressure and bullying.

Treatments

Children and teenagers with eating disorders are often treated with diet, nutritional, and psychological counseling, and medication. Antidepressants are sometimes prescribed by doctors for patients who also suffer from depression. Individual, family, and group therapy may help in uncovering emotional issues, including family conflict or past abuse which may be adding to the problem. The ultimate goal is to deal with underlying issues, return the weight to normal, and help the child progress towards a healthier body image. As with many illnesses, combating an eating disorder requires a team approach using a healthcare provider, possibly specialists, family members to lend support, and the willingness of the person suffering from the illness.

In conclusion, even though African-American children and teenagers are significantly more often overweight than White children and teens, they are usually more comfortable with their body size. This could explain why eating disorders are less common in the African-American community. However, as minority children and teens adopt the body image ideal of mainstream society, they may begin to display the same distorted sense of body image as their mainstream peers. If left untreated, eating disorders can lead to long-term medical and psychological problems that drastically affect one's quality of life.

CHAPTER 4 • EXERCISE A

Use the checklist below to help investigate whether you or someone you love could have an eating disorder. Take it with you to your doctor's visit and share it with him or her. Sometimes, eating disorders go undiagnosed because we are simply not aware of the right questions to ask.

Behaviors
___ Restrict food intake to make me feel more in control
___ Feeling out of control with eating
___ Exercise excessively in order to compensate for the amount of food eaten
___ Self-induced vomiting
___ Temporary fasting in order to make up for food eaten
___ Using drugs to control weight
___ Rituals around food
___ Weighing self often
___ Counting calories

Emotional
___ Depressed
___ Mood swings
___ Guilt about eating
___ Extreme anxiety about becoming fat
___ Poor self-esteem
___ Eating when anxious or upset
___ Shame about eating habits

Psychological

___ Need to be perfect in all activities

___ Preoccupation with food and eating

___ Need for structure

___ Difficulty altering eating schedule

___ Alternating between being in control of eating and totally out of control

___ Trouble concentrating

Social

___ Eats alone often

___ Hides eating habits

___ Avoids friends

___ Strained relationships with friends and family due to food issues

Physical

___ Irregular periods

___ Throat irritation

___ Frequent weight highs and lows

___ Swollen salivary glands

___ Hair loss

___ Puffy cheeks

___ Broken blood vessels under eyes from straining when vomiting

___ Fainting or dizzy spells

___ Tired

___ Tooth or gum disease

CHAPTER 4 • EXERCISE B

Does your child suffer from low self-esteem? Use the questionnaire below to see if your child displays the following behavior:

1. Does your child resist participating in normal social activities such as swimming, slumber parties, etc.?
2. Is your child a loner?
3. Is your child performing poorly in school?
4. Is he or she engaging in risky behavior such as smoking, drug, or alcohol use?
5. Does your child seem depressed?
6. Is your child bullying other kids?

CHAPTER FIVE

The Horrors of the Couch Potato
How Computers, Television, and Video Games Contribute to Childhood Obesity

Objectives

- Understand the influence of television on shaping the dietary habits of children

- Understand the differences in television programming targeting African-American audiences when compared to those targeting the general public

After a long day at work or school, many of us love to end the day by watching our favorite television shows. Not only do we enjoy it, but television can also entertain kids and keep them quiet while we do other tasks around the house or just unwind. How many times has the Disney Channel or Nickelodeon kept your child busy? The Nielsen Media Research is a company that tracks what people watch on TV. It found that most children spend about 6.5 hours a day watching television, using the computer, and playing video games. We know that as viewing increases, so does a child's weight and BMI. This is true regardless of socioeconomic status or ethnicity. This link between screen time (television, computer use and video games) and weight affects all children. However, TV viewing is greater among minority children than White children. The CDC reports that three times as many African-American children and 1.5 times as many Hispanic children watch five or more hours of television per day then White children.

TV is a problem because kids are not active when they watch. In addition, many of the commercials shown on television are for unhealthy foods; the types of food commercials geared towards Black audiences are usually fast food and junk food. These commercials tend to advertise foods high in fat and low in nutrients. Researchers found that food ads aimed at Blacks are almost double the number of food ads aimed at Whites. Black children who watch more television than their White counterpart also eat more unhealthy snacks.

Seeing these commercials on TV, especially during dinner time, may make people crave unhealthy foods more. You can also simply lose track of what you are eating. Have you ever sat down with a new bag of chips to watch your favorite TV show? After a few minutes of watching TV, have you tried to reach for some chips and find none are left? This is known as mindless eating. Eating without even being aware! Our kids do this often.

If you think the commercials are bad, think about some of the TV shows aimed at African Americans. Many of them are likely to show unhealthy foods and characters. Scenes that often focus on typical "soul foods"—fried chicken, macaroni and cheese, and collard greens with ham hocks, are much more common on TV shows aimed at the African-American community. It is estimated that 27% of actors and actresses on African-

TABLE 5.1

Percentage of Commercials in African-American Prime Time

Type of Commercial	Percent of Total Commercials
Fast Foods	31%
Sweets	36%
Cereals and Grains	6%
Chicken/Turkey	1%
Coffee/Tea/Water	1%
Non-Fruit Juice	6%
Soda	13%
Restaurant/Food store	6%
Snacks/Condiments	0%
Alcohol	0%

Source: Tirodkar MA, Jain A. Food Messages on African American Television Shows. Am. J Public Health 2003;(3).

American prime time television were overweight, compared to only 2% on general primetime television.

Although many TV programs show unhealthy foods, few show the harmful effects of obesity, such as high blood pressure, stroke, heart diseases, and diabetes.

Some parents may think that if his or her child is reading a book or playing a game instead of watching television, the child is still not burning calories. But in fact they are burning calories. This is known as your resting metabolism. Resting metabolism is the amount of energy our bodies burn when we do nothing.

Research has shown the resting metabolism rate is actually less when watching television compared to doing some other type of sitting activities. Remember, your metabolic rate is how fast your body uses calories. Activities like reading, drawing, and coloring use more energy than watching TV. These activities also stimulate the brain, which is a good thing for children.

CHAPTER 5 • EXERCISE A

How much time do you and your family spend watching television? Do you know how many commercials you watch each day? Use the table below to record your family's television viewing time. Fill in the time each day, along with the number of commercials and total hours you watched television. Also keep track of the food you eat as you watch your favorite shows.

DAY	Number of Food Commercials	Number of Non-Food Commercials	Total Number of All Commercials	Total Hours Spent Watching TV	Food Eaten During Viewing
SUNDAY					
MONDAY					
TUESDAY					
WEDNESDAY					
THURSDAY					
FRIDAY					
SATURDAY					

Following a week of keeping track of your family's viewing habits, try to make some healthy changes. Try to decrease the amount of television by ninety minutes a week at first. Substitute your child's time with playing outside or involvement in after-school sports programs. Think about not watching television on school nights. Think how much more active the family would be! Try to do some exercise when you watch TV, like doing jumping jacks or push ups during commercials. Have your child do the same. If you find you eat a lot of meals while watching TV, turn the television off during mealtime. Try to limit the types of snacks eaten in front of the television. If there is a need to snack, have only fruits and vegetables available. Pay close attention to the messages portrayed during commercials and see if you notice a difference between the types of commercials on television that target minority viewers compared to the commercials targeting majority viewers. The idea is to get healthy television viewing habits.

CHAPTER SIX

The Aftertaste of Overeating

Objectives

- Become familiar with illnesses associated with overweight and obesity including:

    Type 2 Diabetes
    Heart Disease
    High blood Pressure
    Stroke

- Know what the acceptable healthy ranges are for some of the major illnesses listed

We have talked to parents who think that "as long as my child is happy then his or her weight doesn't matter." We already know that we want to raise happy, healthy kids who feel good about themselves. But we need to take a moment to consider the bad effects that carrying extra weight can have on a child. It may be common for most people to think of diabetes, heart disease, and high blood pressure as illnesses that primarily concern adults, but the truth is our children are also at risk. And if your child is overweight or obese, he or she is at risk as well.

One of the most common illnesses associated with overweight and obesity is Type II diabetes. As we discussed in Chapter 2, carbohydrates provide energy for the body. When we eat carbohydrates, they are broken down into one of the smallest sugars, called glucose. Glucose is then picked up by the blood and taken to every cell in the body. Once the glucose is at the cell, it knocks on the cell's door. A hormone called insulin must be with the blood's sugar to get it in the door of the cell. Once the insulin knocks, the cell easily takes the blood sugar inside. If our cells don't need all the glucose in our blood, our body smartly "stores" the glucose to be used at a later time when the cells may need it. Diabetes occurs when the cells of our body cannot use the glucose in the blood which remains in the blood, causing high blood sugar levels. As physicians, we like to check blood sugar levels when a person has not eaten for at least eight hours. This is known as a "fasting" blood sugar. If it is less than 100 mg/dL, then it is considered normal. If it is 100–125, then it is pre-diabetes. If it is over 126 mg/dL, it is highly suspicious for diabetes.

There are two types of Diabetes, Type I and Type II. In Type 1 (insulin-dependent diabetes), the body is unable to make insulin. Once the glucose gets to the cell door, there is no insulin to help get it in.

Insulin is made by an organ in the body called the pancreas. For people with Type I diabetes, they suddenly stop making insulin without any reason. Although we are not sure why this happens, it usually only happens to children. In fact it used to be called juvenile onset diabetes. People with Type I diabetes must take insulin for their entire life since their bodies do not make insulin. It happens randomly and usually does not run in families.

Type II Diabetes happens when the body is able to make insulin but the cells do not respond to insulin as well as they used to. It takes a lot more insulin to knock on the cell's door to get the same blood sugar in. The body then has to make more and more insulin to help the glucose get inside of the cell. Again this causes blood sugar levels to be high. We are not sure exactly why this happens, but we do know that being overweight or obese makes it much more likely that a person will get Type II diabetes. This is the diabetes that older people usually get. In fact it used to be called "adult onset diabetes"; this is no longer true. Although the exact number is not known, it is believed that a significant percentage of all new diabetes cases among young people is due to Type II Diabetes. Type II diabetes is more common in African Americans, Native Americans, and Mexican Americans than Whites. We also know that it can run in families. Unfortunately, children as young as ten can have Type II diabetes. People with this kind of diabetes can manage it with good eating habits, exercising, medicine, and/or insulin.

Obesity and Type II diabetes are clearly linked. A lifestyle with little physical activity and a high-fat calorie-rich diet all contribute to the recent increase of childhood overweight and Type II diabetes. One of the main reasons for this is the overall eating habits of children have changed drastically. We know that currently most children eat too much fat (and hence calories), salt and cholesterol than recommended. A higher percentage of fat is eaten by African-American and Hispanic girls and African-American boys than White boys or girls. This can be one of the reasons that African-American and Hispanic children are suffering from overweight and diabetes more than White children.

Type II diabetes can be a manageable long term disease. However, if not managed, Type II diabetes can have bad outcomes. If the blood sugar is not controlled for years, serious problems can occur which can interfere with a normal way of life. Often, especially in the early stages, the diabetic person will show no symptoms, although increased thirst, frequent urination, and weight loss may be early signs. One of the signs that the body has high insulin levels (but not necessarily high blood sugar) is darkening of the skin on the cheeks, neck, and sometime in the armpits or genital area. This darkening is known as *acanthosis nigricans* and it occurs more often in people of color. Although they do not have symptoms, the high blood sugar levels are still damaging the body. Constantly high blood sugar levels can cause blindness, heart disease, stroke, kidney damage, and nerve damage. People who have diabetes for a long time (ten to twenty years) may lose their vision, have limbs removed or need to be on dialysis (a machine that cleans the blood because the kidneys are too damaged to clean it properly). If young people start to get diabetes, they may have some of these bad outcomes in their thirties and forties. This is when people are in the prime of their life, often responsible for families.

The good news about Type II diabetes is that it can be prevented or delayed with a healthy diet and daily exercise. Eating a diet rich in whole grains instead of simple sugars and getting regular exercise can greatly improve your child's odds of remaining diabetes free. Unfortunately, many people find it hard to make these changes. That's why it is so important to develop good habits early in life. Parents play a very important role in promoting good eating habits in their children. Eating right not only helps your child now but also forms life-long habits that will help prevent illnesses later.

Another common illness associated with overweight and obesity is heart disease. The heart pumps blood throughout the body. It uses a "roadway," or arteries, to pump blood away from the heart and veins that return blood to the heart. The goal is for the heart to get blood to all of the body's vital organs. Blood delivers oxygen and food to the cells in the vital organs so that they can function and grow properly. As people get older, the heart and arteries can become weaker from years of unhealthy living. Anything that can cause damage to the heart or arteries is known as heart disease. According to the CDC, heart disease is the leading cause of death in the United States.

Children usually have nice, strong, healthy hearts that can easily pump blood throughout the body. The arteries are strong yet flexible, making blood easy to flow through them. But what happens when our heart is not as strong as it should be? What happens if our arteries become hard and stiff?

Have you ever turned on your faucet and the water goes very slow down the drain. Maybe there is build–up of junk in the pipes. Most of us rely on products that will unclog the pipe or you may call a plumber. Well imagine if your arteries became clogged. As we get older, our arteries can become clogged with fatty streaks, cell waste, cholesterol, and other junk. The junk can build up and form larger piles of junk known as plaque. This process of build up in the arteries is known as *atherosclerosis*. Once atherosclerosis sets in, it is much harder for blood to get through the vessels. Your heart has to work even harder to get the blood to the vital organs.

FIGURE 7

Clogged Artery

Decreased blood flow to heart may cause heart muscle damage

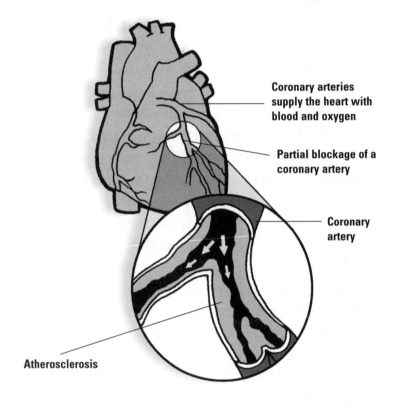

Coronary arteries supply the heart with blood and oxygen

Partial blockage of a coronary artery

Coronary artery

Atherosclerosis

Coronary arteries progressively closing (from left to right) resulting from coronary artery disease.

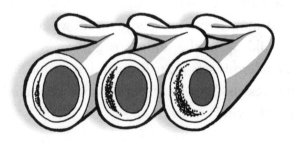

In the past, plaque build-up was typically seen mainly in older Americans, but now we think this process is starting at much earlier ages because of bad diets, lack of exercise, and obesity.

One of the main causes of clogged arteries is high cholesterol levels. We recommend people have their cholesterol levels checked, especially overweight children and those with a strong family history of high cholesterol. Your healthcare provider will be able to determine how often you and your child should be checked and whether you are at risk. We have covered the importance of maintaining good levels of cholesterol in Chapter Two. Take the time to review the information again. It is important for parents to understand that high LDL cholesterol, high triglycerides and fatty streak and plaque build up can start in childhood. This process does not have symptoms, which means children do not appear to be ill. However, as they grow older the problem gets worse and can lead to even more serious heart disease. For children 2–19, an acceptable level of fasting total cholesterol is less than 170 mg/dL, borderline is 170–199 mg/dL, and high is greater than 200 mg/dL. Triglycerides should be less than 150 mg/dL, and HDL (good guys) should be at least 35 mg/dL.

High blood pressure or hypertension can also be associated with overweight and obesity. As arteries become more and more stiff, the heart has to work harder and harder to push blood through the arteries. Imagine water in a water hose that is barely dripping. We would say that is "low pressure." Now imagine a fire truck water hose at full blast, spraying a lot of water very fast with a lot of force. We would say that is "high pressure." The heart does something similar. As the arteries get smaller and smaller from the build up of plaque, the heart has to pump harder to keep the same amount of blood to vital organs. This increase in the force of the heart pump is known as high blood pressure, or hypertension. Although it is good that the heart is able to work harder, the extra pressure on the vital organs can cause damage. Blood pressure is recorded with two numbers; the top number is the pressure the heart uses when it is pumping blood and the bottom number is the pressure the heart uses when it is at rest. For normal, healthy adults, blood pressure should be less than 120/80. Since children are growing and are generally a lot smaller than adults, their normal blood pressure will depend on their age, gender, and height, so we can not use absolute cut off numbers like we do for adults. However for older children, if the blood pressure is greater than 120/80 it may be cause for concern because that is higher than what is acceptable for adults. You should check with your child's doctor to determine if your child's blood pressure is okay.

Some people don't experience any symptoms that indicate the heart is pumping harder, while others may have headaches or may frequently feel tired. High blood pressure has been called the "silent killer" because many who have it do not know they are affected. People with long standing high blood pressure that goes untreated can develop strokes, blindness, and kidney failure, as well as other serious illnesses such as heart disease. It can also lead to death.

We have noticed an increase of high blood pressure in children. In one study, 11% of obese children had repeated high blood pressure on three separate occasions and the risk of getting high blood pressure was three times greater among overweight children compared to normal weight children. These statistics are alarming. If children get high blood pressure at young ages, it can lead to strokes, heart attacks, and blindness in their twenties and thirties.

Heart disease, high cholesterol levels, and high blood pressure can damage the heart so much that they can cause the heart to stop working properly. This is clinically known as a heart attack. All of the problems can also cause bleeding into the brain, which is known as a stroke. Overweight children who grow up to become overweight adults have a greater risk for heart attacks, heart failure, and chest pain from problems that start in childhood.

The good news about heart disease is that much of it can be prevented or improved with good nutrition, just like diabetes. However, heart disease can occur without symptoms for many years; thus people may not realize they have a problem. This is where parents play a major role. If you can get your child in the habit of eating well, getting physical activity, and maintaining a normal weight, you can help them prevent major heart disease later in life. If our children continue on the current path, we will have more children with high blood pressure, clogged arteries, and possibly heart attacks and strokes than ever before.

There are other unexpected illnesses associated with overweight and obesity, such as different types of cancer, sleep apnea, and asthma. There is a proven link between adult obesity and certain forms of cancer; the jury is still out on a link with childhood forms of cancer. However, there is a link between overweight adolescents and breast cancer. Girls who gain more than twenty pounds beginning at eighteen years through midlife are twice as likely to develop breast cancer after menopause compared to those whose weight remain constant.

There are other potential side effects to consider as a result of being overweight or obese. Because carrying added weight is part of one's appearance, it may be common to forget about the underlying effects being overweight and obese has on a person.

Remember, we have touched on the psychological issues associated with being overweight. But you may not realize that being overweight or obese also has an effect on us when our bodies are supposed to be resting. This condition is called sleep apnea. Obstructive sleep apnea is a condition in which a person stops breathing during sleep. The brain kind of acts like an alarm clock on snooze and continuously wakes up the person so that they will breathe. This can happen hundreds of times during the night, reducing the amount of sleep which is essential for a healthy body. If sleep apnea is considerably bad, the person may stop breathing altogether and die in his or her sleep.

One of the main causes of obstructive sleep apnea is obesity. When lying down there can be a lot of weight on the airway, which can cause the airway to close. The airway is a tube located in the neck; it connects your mouth and nose to your lungs. If people have bad sleep apnea, they may have to sleep with special machines to make sure they breathe throughout the night. A telltale sign of sleep apnea are kids who snore very loudly then have periods of quietness (10–20 seconds) with the abrupt restarting of loud snoring. While weight loss can sometimes be beneficial in decreasing obstructive sleep apnea, overweight children are still more likely to experience sleep disturbances serious enough to require surgical correction.

In addition to sleep apnea, there is also a strong association between childhood overweight, asthma, and asthma severity. The signs and symptoms of asthma such as shortness of breath, wheezing, coughing, and chest tightness result when the small airways in the lungs are extra sensitive to certain triggers. The airways in asthmatic children are frequently sensitive to cigarette smoke, animals, automobile exhaust, and allergens such as pollen and ragweed. In addition to airway narrowing, the walls become swollen and fluid builds up within the airways. The once normally open airway is now narrow and blocked. It is as if you attempted to drink a thick milk shake through a coffee stirrer instead of a straw. A once easy practice becomes strained and very difficult. We are still not sure which comes first—the asthma or obesity. Perhaps the overweight is linked to a lack of physical activity that many asthmatics avoid, as exercise often worsens asthmatic symptoms. Perhaps the sleep disturbances experienced by many overweight children set up the airways to be hypersensitive. What is clear is that overweight children have nearly double the risk of developing asthma.

To sum it all up, the destruction caused by an inactive lifestyle and improper nutrition go far beyond the physical appearance of obesity. We now know that most of the life-threatening illnesses discussed in this chapter are no longer reserved for adults but are now being diagnosed at an alarming rate in children. Take action now to gain a healthier lifestyle for you and your child. Get out there and start moving.

CHAPTER 6 • EXERCISE A

Know you and your child's numbers

1. If you or your child has a fasting blood sugar taken, what should your blood sugar be to be considered normal?
2. What level is highly suggestive of diabetes in both children and adults?
3. What is considered a normal blood pressure for adults? For children?
5. You and your child's fasting total cholesterol should be less than what number?
6. When is the last time you or your child has had a complete physical to check the items discussed in this chapter?

CHAPTER 6 • EXERCISE B

Could you or your child have the early warning signs of Type II diabetes? Use the checklist below to see if you or your child displays the following symptoms and/or signs.

Type II Diabetes Symptoms
1. Excessive thirst
2. Frequent urination
3. Excessive hunger
4. Rapid or sudden weight loss
5. Tiredness and fatigue
6. Irritability
7. Sores that take a long time to heal
8. Dry itchy skin
9. Blurry eyesight
10. Unexplained rashes

CHAPTER SEVEN

Exercise
Who needs it?

Objectives

- Understanding the role of energy use in the body
- Examining the barriers to consistent physical activity
- Understanding why physical activity is important to health
- How to build a plan: tips to get your child moving

If your child's doctor has told you that you need to increase your child's physical activity because he or she is overweight or obese, and your doctor has also recommended that you become more physically active even though you are not overweight, you're probably wondering what to do next. Gym memberships can be expensive, we know, but that doesn't mean you cannot be active. Most research has found that the key to maintaining a healthy weight is not only eating right, but also becoming physically active. By understanding the role of physical activity in improving your child's health you will be ready to take your family on a journey of healthy living.

Physical activity can help in maintaining a healthy weight or losing extra weight. We have already discussed that energy is needed to make the body work. The body uses energy for everything, even when you are resting or sleeping. All parts of our body—including the heart, muscles, brain and all of the organs—use energy. This is known as Basic Energy Use (BEU). Any activity that you do over these basic functions is called Active Energy Use (AEU). We have AEU when we are awake. This includes activities like walking, talking, reading, etc. Even watching our children play soccer requires extra energy. (The brain has to process and interpret what you see and hear.) If you add up your BEU and AEU, then that equals your TEU, or total energy use. Increasing your TEU will help the body use extra energy, which helps to burn fat. Your BEU remains pretty much the same unless you build muscle. Muscle uses more energy than fat.

Children should get at least 60 minutes of physical activity every day! This activity should be moderate or vigorous, which means the activity should cause an increase in breathing and heart rate. This may seem like a lot to some, but it really is not. Physical activity is anything that increases your child's heart rate and breathing rate and makes them feel like they are working. Some simple examples are housework, walking briskly, jogging, cheerleading, and playing sports. And don't forget about dancing! (At no time should your child complain of dizziness, chest pain or extreme pain. **If they do, they should stop immediately**.) Your child's AEU for a specific activity depends on your child's fitness level, age, gender, and intensity. Older kids are usually stronger than younger kids and boys more than girls. It is helpful for children when families do physical activities together. You can participate in family activities like walking, bike riding, playing in the park, or dancing. Remember, this is not a sprint, so no need to overdue it. Start slowly and work your way up to 60 minutes. (See "How to get started" at the end of the chapter.)

Let's face it; we live in an instant world; we expect everything to happen right now. Modern conveniences have been wonderful. Think how life would be if we did not have cars, microwaves, washing machines, or computers. Imagine if children had to walk everywhere they went. Well technology is a double–edged sword. While it has the potential to make our life much easier, it has also actually made our life much more difficult to schedule daily activity. Even our children's curriculums have contributed to the lack of physical activity. According to the CDC, inactivity is twice as common among females (14%) as males (7%) and among Black females (21%) as White females (12%).

Unfortunately, individuals at increased risk of having low levels of physical activity are children from ethnic minorities (especially girls) in the preadolescent/adolescent age groups, children living in poverty, children with disabilities, children residing in apartments or public housing, and children living in neighborhoods where outdoor physical activity is restricted by climate, safety concerns, and/or lack of facilities.

No More Excuses

Many of us can think of five quick reasons why we cannot exercise or allow our children to exercise. As physicians we have heard them all. However, we cannot allow these road blocks to keep us from saving our lives and the lives of our children. So let's discuss a few concerns and what you can do to get over the hurdles.

Safety is often a major concern when it comes to physical activity, especially for people who live in high crime areas. Oftentimes mothers may not think that neighborhoods are safe enough to let children go outside without supervision. Parents may fear that their child will fall victim to crime or be pressured to commit crime (peer pressure). Because parents may work, children may be left home during the hours after school. If kids cannot go outside, this significantly limits play time.

We understand that **location** plays a major role in access to a child's physical activity as well. Urban areas tend to have more sidewalks than suburban and rural areas, which is contributing to the southeastern region of the United States having some of the highest rates of obesity overall. If you live in an urban area and do not have outdoor access, you can do a series of jumping jacks, arm windmills, or play games like Jacks, Twister, or Pictionary. Anything that requires some movement is helpful.

Although it may seem strange, hair may also be a barrier to exercise. We speak from personal experience. African-American girls are the most physically inactive and overweight of any group. Some of this can be contributed to the fact that Black girls do not want to mess up their hair. It is vital that we get our girls to move. We have some tips at the end of the chapter to help your daughters. As parents you should strive to reinforce health as your family's main interest, for when you are healthy you automatically look and feel better.

You may be thinking, "This all sounds good, but what happens to my child while in school? Shouldn't there be some physical activity there?" While you may be correct in thinking that

the schools should have physical education as part of the curriculum, the truth is some may not. The percentage of students
who attend a daily physical education class dropped from 42% in
1991 to 28% in 2003. There has been a lot of TV coverage about
the lack of physical activity among American children. Federal
programs like the No Child Left Behind Act, which took effect
in 2001, have caused many schools across the country to scale
back on time spent in physical activity in favor of more time
spent in the classroom. Many health officials believe that,
increasingly, less time will be allotted for physical activity, or
even recess. Across the nation, fewer physical education classes
have been offered in schools since the act went into effect. In
2006, the National Association for Sport and Physical Education
and the American Heart Association released a report entitled
*2006 Shape of the nation report: Status of Physical Education in the
USA*. According to the report, nearly a third of states do not
mandate physical education for elementary and middle school
students, and twelve states allow students to earn required physical education credits through online physical education courses.
In 2005, the CDC asked hundreds of students about their physical activity habits as part of the National Youth Risk Behavior
Survey (YRBS). Only 33 percent of all high school students said
they had gym class everyday and 56 percent reported playing on
one or more team.

    As physicians concerned with the dramatic increase in child-
hood overweight and its associated illnesses, we believe that
physical education should be a core subject because its presence
in a child's life has just as much bearing on life outcomes as pass-
ing a standardized test. Physical activities as part of the school
curriculum promotes good health, friendship, partnership, and a

healthy level of competition. Recently, a thirteen-member panel of medical experts reviewed 850 scientific papers and studies on children and the benefits of physical activity. After very careful study, they found that regular moderate to vigorous exercise three to five times per week was effective in:

- Controlling weight
- Helping to reduce weight
- Reducing blood pressure
- Raising HDL ("good") cholesterol
- Reducing the risk of diabetes and some forms of cancer
- Improving psychological well-being, including gaining more self-confidence and higher self-esteem
- Improving academic performance.

Maintaining a healthy weight is important, but being physically active with or without major weight loss adds benefits to our health and well-being.

So, Let's Get Moving

Now that we have talked about physical activity, let's build a custom plan for your child. First, let's pick a time of day that your child can participate in physical activity. This time may change depending on the time of year and you and your child's schedule. Ideally you should set aside 60–90 minutes. Remember it may take some time to set up and clean up. Start with exercising three times per week and work your child up to at least five times a week.

An easy activity for most children and their family is walking. Walking can be an easy, fun, and cheap way to get physical activity. You and your child can walk 30–60 minutes at one time or you can split the time up. For example, you and your child may walk for 20 minutes in the morning and then 20 minutes in the afternoon. And don't forget the walking that you and your child may do throughout the day. A great way to keep up with how much you walk is to get a pedometer. A pedometer is a small electronic device (usually about the size of a pager) that clips onto your belt or pants. It counts all of the steps you take. Your child should put it on first thing in the morning and keep it on all day. Your child can check how many steps they have taken throughout the day. Both healthy children and adults should aim for "10,000" steps a day. If your child is not getting 10,000 steps, they can try to increase their walking throughout the day. Pedometers can be found where exercise clothing and equipment are sold.

Now, let's pick an activity. You know your family's resources best and can choose an appropriate activity based on your child's age and financial resources. For young children, ages 4–8, try to pick "free" play time. This is unstructured time for you to play with your child at the park or a safe room in your home. The goal is to keep your child moving and laughing.

For children ages 8–12 and teenagers, try to figure what they like to do for fun. Children who participate in activities that they like are more likely to continue. They may be ready to participate in organized sports. Check your neighborhood for youth clubs (like the Boys and Girls Clubs of America), local recreation centers operated by your city or county, or private centers.

For example, there may be reasonably-priced dance groups or martial arts classes located near you. Older children can also exercise to DVDs. These are often lower cost (less than $20) and can be done in the privacy of the teenagers' home if they do not want to exercise in public. It is also an option for parents who are concerned about safe neighborhoods. One of our favorite (and cheapest) forms of exercising is dancing. Your child can find one hour a day to turn on their favorite radio (or TV video) station and practice the latest dance moves. This can be fun for the entire family. You can have dance contests to see who knows all the latest moves.

All of the recommendations provided hare are suggestions. Remember, you should have your child examined by his or her doctor before beginning an exercise program.

Below are several ideas for fun and games with your family. Try some of these fun exercises at home with your kids. Try and do them for at least 30–60 minutes a day.

1. Play Simon Says using jumping jacks, skips, or other physical moves.
2. Have a fast-walking race and see who wins.
3. Take a bike ride together.
4. Use dance video games such as Dance Dance Revolution®.
5. Make up some new dance moves.
6. Have a timed scavenger hunt.
7. Go to the park.
8. Walk around the inside of a mall at least five times.
9. Walk 10,000 steps a day.

Whichever activity you decide to do with your child, aim to do it three times a week, then work your child up to at least five times a week for 60 minutes per day. Stretch for at least five minutes before any activity to make sure your muscles are warm and five minutes afterwards to cool down. (Examples of stretching is trying to reach your arms and legs out as far as they will go comfortably and moving the trunk of your body in a circle.)

If your child is going to be walking or running, we recommend proper athletic shoes. Clothing should be loose and comfortable. For teenaged girls, they also need a good sports bra if they are engaging in moderate or vigorous activity. Many teenage girls are concerned about the effects of sweating on the hair. If this is the case, they can pin or wrap their hair before exercising, with a sweat band around the hair line. Another option is for her to pull her hair back in a pony tail or braid the hair. She may have to experiment a few times, but hairstyles should not stop young women from being physically active.

Once the time and activity are chosen, keep track of your daily activity. For your younger children, you can keep this information as a chart. Older kids can keep exercise diaries.

CHAPTER 7• EXERCISE A

Exercise Planning

1. Determine with your child's physician how long your child should exercise and how many times a week?
2. Determine some examples of physical activity that your child enjoy?
3. Understand the benefits of exercise besides weight loss?
4. List at least three different one hour periods (day and time) that your child could exercise?

CHAPTER EIGHT

Move It, Lose It, and Love It for Life

Objectives

- Incorporate what we've learned into a healthy weight loss plan for overweight children
- Making a lifestyle change beginning with eating habits

Because children are constantly growing, we NEVER recommend fad diets or any type of diet pills to help children lose weight. These can be very dangerous to children and have side effects that we may not even know about yet. We think all children should follow the healthy guidelines that we have outlined in our book so far. However, we do know that for some children who are overweight or obese or who have medical problems because of their weight, a diet may be recommended to lose weight.

When attempting to achieve weight loss, it is important to keep in mind that any weight-loss diet should be low in calories only, not in essential nutrients. Nutrients are important for growth and development in children. If neglected, as a result of extreme and unhealthy dieting, a child's overall health can be compromised. Carefully cut down on the amount of fat and calories in your family's diet and refrain from placing your child on a restrictive diet. Replace unhealthy eating habits with better alternatives. Even with extremely overweight children, weight loss should be gradual. Healthy eating should be viewed as a lifestyle change and not merely a temporary shift in behavior. Weight lost during a diet is frequently regained unless children are motivated to change their eating habits and increase their activity levels. Weight control through healthy eating and physical activity must be considered a lifelong effort and works best if the entire family is involved. Children should be active in their health management and have a voice. And, parents should be supportive and provide options for some unhealthy behaviors such as limiting trips to a fast food restaurant. Or, allow children to order what they want but tell them it has to be from the kid's menu—then you do the same! Introduce these changes slowly. Model the behavior that you want your child to have. Children frequently imitate their parents. Healthy changes should be made for the entire family. However, any weight management program for your child should be supervised by a physician.

Where to Start?

To help your child lose weight, we recommend you start at the doctor's office. Given what we already know about the numerous health risks of being overweight, we cannot stress enough that all children should have annual checkups with their doctors. To be certain you are on the right track, bring these questions to your child's checkup and review them with the doctor:

- Is my child overweight, or obese?
- Could my child's overall health be at risk because of the extra weight?
- Is it safe for my child to begin a slow weight loss program? If so, what do you recommend?

If the doctor has determined that your child should begin a weight management program, discuss whether starting with a calorie reducing program will work best. If children expend more calories than they consume, they will lose weight. Remember 3,500 calories is roughly equal to one pound of fat. If you reduce your child's daily calorie intake by 500, he or she can accomplish a one pound per week weight loss.

Revisit Chapter 2 to see how many calories your child needs each day based on age, gender, and activity level. Next, use the food and exercise logs at the end of this book (make copies first) to determine what your child eats and what exercises your child does in an average week. You can then look at it and see ways to make changes based on what you have learned in this book. Is your child eating too many calories? Are the extra calories from high calorie foods or are the portion sizes too big? Does your child get enough physical activity? Does he/she get three to five hours per week at least (the goal is one hour per day)? Here are some practical tips to help you and your child cut calories:

Water

What your child drinks is probably the first thing you should try to change. Our bodies are mainly made of water. The body needs water for everything we do. Both children and adults need a lot of water every day. Your child should drink about eight cups of water a day. They should reach for water when they are thirsty but also throughout the day even when they are not thirsty. This will help them maintain hydration and will also cut down on hunger. Water can fill up your stomach and keep it from being empty. A good way to tell if your child is getting enough water is to look at the urine. Urine should be only slightly yellow, almost clear. This indicates that your child is very well hydrated and has good water intake.

Cut the Sugar—Sweetened Beverages (Juice, Soda, Etc.)

We've already talked about carbohydrates and sugar in the diet in Chapter 2, but we have not specifically talked about sugar in juice, soda and other beverages. Many parents believe juice is a great addition to their children's diet. Oftentimes when we ask parents if they give their children juice, they enthusiastically reply, "of course". And some children drink sodas two to three times a day. Many people are not aware how all the calories in sodas and juice add up. Most juices have about 120 calories in eight ounces. Juices and soda in the 20–oz. bottle usually have 300 calories per bottle! If your child is drinking five or six cups of juice a day (or two 20–oz. bottles) that can be an extra 600 calories a day! Merely cutting the amount of regular juice and sodas can save your child many calories in one day. While many juices may have added vitamins and mineral, it is much healthier to eat the fruit instead of drinking the juice. We recommend no more than eight ounces of juice (100% juice is best) a day and no sodas. You can cut down on juice and soda gradually by:

- Mixing half water, half juice to start
- Buying fruit-flavored water
- Trying zero calorie juices and sodas
- Reducing the amount of juice and soda purchased for the home.

Vegetables and Fruits

There is no such thing as too many fruits and vegetables. We like fresh fruits and vegetables, but know sometimes they may go bad if we keep them too long. You can also use frozen and canned fruits and vegetables if this is the case. Children should have access to vegetables and fruits throughout the day to snack on. Aim for "five-a-day" as an easy way to remember.

Milk and Dairy Products

Milk and dairy products are a good source of calcium. Many children like foods such as milk, cheese, ice cream and yogurt. If your child is older than two, then he or she can have low fat or skimmed milk. We also like low fat yogurt as a good source of calcium. They also have lower fat cheeses and ice creams. Children can eat 2–3 servings of dairy products a day. Consider giving your child a glass of low fat chocolate milk with breakfast. Try giving your child a slice of lower fat cheese on a sandwich or a small yogurt at lunchtime. These are all great ideas to get dairy products in your child's diet.

Meals

Remember meals should be low fat. Each day should start with breakfast; this provides energy for the morning. Lunch and dinner should have a protein (meat, beans, eggs, and nuts), a whole grain starch, and vegetable or fruit. Meats should be lean and preferably baked, boiled, or broiled without skin. Children should eat off of small plates (10" diameter or less) with the right sized portion. Half the plate should be vegetables or fruits, a quarter should be protein, and a quarter should be starch. If your child asks for seconds, try to start with the veggies and fruits first. Also, it is OK for children to drink water while eating.

Junk Food and Sweets

Just as juice and soda can add a lot of extra calories to your child's diet, so can junk food! Now everyone may like a treat once in a while, but daily consumption of junk food can lead to problems down the road. If your child is eating junk food more than one to two times a week or is eating a large amount at one time, then it is too much. Stress to your child that junk food is for special times (weekends, celebrations, etc.) and not for every day. Next, look at what junk food your child likes and think about how you can change that to a healthier alternative. For example, if they like potato chips, maybe they could try baked potato chips or only eat a very small bag. If you buy the larger bag, try splitting it up into small plastic bags and give your child only a small plastic bag as a snack. If they like cakes and cookies, try to give them one small snack cake or three to four small cookies. Again, you should only have these foods on weekends or special occasions.

Better yet, look for low calorie and fat recipes for snacks and let your child help you make them. You could make some snacks and perhaps share the rest with friends and family.

Extra Vitamins and Minerals

We do not routinely suggest vitamin and minerals for children, but if they are on a weight loss program, they may benefit from a daily multivitamin. This will ensure that they do not miss any important vitamins and minerals. We recommend you speak with your child's doctor before giving him or her vitamins.

Keeping Track

Now that you know how to make changes, let's revisit the food/exercise log. Incorporate the changes slowly into your child's diet (aim for one change every one to two weeks) and see how the log changes over time. Depending on your family's habits, it may take several months to make all the necessary changes. Remember this is a marathon, not a sprint. Families that make changes slowly are more likely to stick to them.

Healthy eating and regular physical activity are key components for physical and mental well-being. By establishing these habits early in life, many diseases associated with obesity can be avoided. One of the most effective methods of achieving this goal is to model these behaviors for our children. By setting an example and demonstrating a commitment to healthy eating and routine physical exercise, children will naturally incorporate these behaviors into their daily activities. Establishing healthy eating and promoting physical activity can enhance the overall health of your family.

Final Exercise

So now you have read all about overweight and obesity and have been given tips throughout the book to deal with them, let's make a plan to get healthier.

1. First, let us determine the extent of the overweight problem in your family. Visit Chapter One to determine if your child or other family members are overweight.

2. Let's make our house health friendly. Remember, do the exercise at the end of Chapter Two to determine if we have healthy foods in our pantry. When going to the grocery store, let's try not to get junk food or soda and limit the juice. Remember to look at food labels and try to avoid high fat, high salt, and high calorie foods. Try to pick out fruits and vegetables (fresh, frozen or, as a last resort, canned). Try to limit meats with skin or cuts of meat that are high in calories. If you are not sure about items, ask your local supermarket manager.

3. Review the "Healthy Tips" and the exercise at the end of Chapter Three. This will give you practical tips for the real world. Pay special attention to the "Healthy Grocery Store" checklist. Try to eat five to six small meals a day (keeping in mind not to exceed calorie requirements). Remember it is OK to split "one" meal in halves, thirds, or quarters and eat it later if it is big. Skip the sodas and juice and replace them with water (regular or flavored).

4. Keep track of your child's and family TV viewing habits. Review the exercise you've completed at the end of Chapter Five and think about how TV influences your choices. Try to limit TV viewing and computer time to no more than two hours total. Also, make a rule of no eating in front of the TV.

5. Remember, while we want to encourage health, we don't want to encourage low self-esteem. Reassess your child to make sure he or she is happy and has a sense of selfworth. Make sure you praise your child for all accomplishments and achievements and reassure them that you love them unconditionally.

6. If your child is overweight, could they have another disease? It is always good to have an annual physical for your child. This is a good time to discuss your child's weight, abnormal symptoms they may complain of, and any family history that might be important. Your child's doctor can further discuss your child's weight status and risk for disease.

7. MAKE SURE YOU HAVE FUN!

8. Pick out a physical activity that you and your family can do most days of the week for at least 30 -60 minutes. Remember it can be formal exercise (such as after-school sports) or informal (walking, running, bike riding, dancing to the radio, pre-recorded exercise DVDs). The key is to figure out what exercise is going to work for your family.

9. WRITE DOWN WHAT YOU DO. Use a food/exercise diary to keep track of your habits and weight if needed. (See the example at the end of this chapter.) People who

Weekly Food Log

	Breakfast	Lunch	Dinner	Snacks	Exercise
Monday					
Tuesday					
Wednesday					
Thursday					
Friday					
Saturday					
Sunday					

write down what they eat and what they do are more successful at achieving and maintaining a healthy weight.
You can review the diary at the end of the week and look
to see how you can improve your child's habits.

Glossary of Terms

Acanthosis Nigricans: Darkening of the skin on the cheeks, neck and sometime in the armpits or genital area which indicates that the body has high insulin levels.

Active Energy Use (AEU): Any energy requirements beyond basic function such as walking, talking, or reading.

Amino Acid: Individual building blocks which make up proteins.

Anorexia Nervosa: A disorder where a person refuses to keep his or her weight anywhere near normal for their height and age.

Asthma: Lung condition that causes shortness of breath, wheezing, coughing, and chest tightness.

Atherosclerosis: Build-up of plaques and debris in the arteries.

Basal Metabolic Rate (BMR): Minimum number of calories needed to keep the body functioning.

Basic Energy Use (BEU): Basic energy requirements for the body to function, such as eating and sleeping.

Body Mass Index (BMI): Measurement scale that health professionals use to estimate the amount of excess weight in the body.

Bone Density: Measures bone hardness.

Bulimia: A psychological disorder characterized by eating an excessive amount of food (commonly known as binging), and then purging by throwing up, exercising excessively, or taking laxatives.

Calorie/kilocalorie: A measure of energy expenditure. You may also see the word "kilocalorie" (kcal) in books and articles on nutrition, diet, or exercise. Simply put, one kilocalorie is equal to 3,500 units of food energy, which is equal to one pound of body weight. If you need to lose one pound, you will need to burn 3,500 units of energy.

Carbohydrates: Provide most of the energy we need in our daily lives. They come from starchy plants and grains such as oat, wheat, barley, and even corn.

Cardio-Respiratory Fitness (also called aerobic endurance or aerobic fitness): A measurement of the body's circulatory and respiratory system's ability to supply fuel and oxygen during physical activity.

Cholesterol: Soft, waxy substance that circulates in the bloodstream and is a component of all your body's cells.

Compulsive Overeating: A psychological disorder otherwise known as binge eating which is strongly linked to obesity. Compulsive overeaters will eat more than 2,500 calories in one sitting or in less than two hours.

Dehydration: Occurs when the body does not receive enough fluids.

Diabetes: A condition in which the cell in the body is not able to use glucose, leading to high blood sugar levels. There is Type I, in which the body doesn't make insulin (hormone needed to get glucose in the cell). Type II diabetes occurs when the body's cells become resistant to insulin. Type II diabetes is usually associated with overweight.

Essential Amino Acids: Nine amino acids that are not produced by the body. You must eat them.

Fat: Stored energy in the body. Keeps the body warm, provides cushioning and insulation for vital internal organs, and helps keep the skin soft.

Food Insecurities: A psychological condition in which a person fears they won't have enough to eat.

Genes: Genetic material passed on by both parents to children.

Glucose: Simple sugar that gives cells energy.

High–Density Lipoprotein (HDL): Also known as good cholesterol because it takes cholesterol away from the blood.

Household Physical Activity: Physical activity which includes (but is not limited to) activities such as sweeping floors, scrubbing, washing windows, and raking the lawn.

Hydrogenation: Process that turns natural liquid oils to a solid at room temperature.

Hypercholesterolemia: Another name for high cholesterol. A high level of cholesterol in the blood.

Hypertension: Another name for high blood pressure. The heart uses higher than normal pressure to pump blood throughout the body.

Leisure-time Physical Activity: Physical activities such as exercise, sports, recreation, or hobbies that are not associated with activities as part of one's regular job, household, or transportation.

Lipoproteins: Special carriers in the body which transport fat to and from cells.

Low-density lipoprotein (LDL): Also known as bad cholesterol because it carries cholesterol to the blood stream.

Malnutrition: Occurs when the body is not getting enough vitamins, minerals, and nutrients to keep the tissues and organs healthy.

The Standard Metabolic Equivalent (MET): A unit of measurement used to estimate the amount of oxygen used by the body during physical activity.

Metabolism: How quickly your body burns calories.

Minerals: An element that aids the body in carrying out it's functions. Commonly found in soil and water.

Moderate-Intensity Physical Activity: Physical activity or exercise that requires a moderate level of effort. Moderate exercise should result in an increase in breathing or heart rate. A slow jog is an example of moderate physical activity.

Monounsaturated Fats: Fats found in nuts, avocadoes, and oils such as olive, peanut, and canola.

National Health and Nutrition Examination Survey (NHANES): A national study of a random sample of U.S. adult and children conducted by the CDC. The study measures a lot of health information on people, including heights and weights.

National Youth Risk Behavior Survey (YRBS): A survey about the physical activity habits of youth conducted in 2005 by the CDC.

Nutrition Label: Lists the ingredients and the nutritional content of packaged foods.

Obese: Body Mass Index measurement above 30 for adults or above the 95th percentile for age and gender for children.

Obstructive Sleep Apnea: A condition in which a person stops breathing during sleep and is then awakening to start breathing again. This cycle can occur hundreds of times during one night.

Organized Physical Activity: Physical activity, such as basketball, baseball, or other organized sports, with an organized group that has a coach, instructor, or leader.

Osteoporosis: Decrease in bone mineral density.

Overweight: Body Mass Index measurement above 25 for adults or between the 85th and 95th percentile for gender and age for children.

Percent Daily Value: Written as "%DV" on the food label, the percentage of nutrients supplied in one serving of food if you were aiming to eat 2,000 calories a day.

Percentile: Simply refers to the percentage of children whose BMI is less than a particular number.

Polyunsaturated Fat: Includes essential fatty acids that the body cannot make. They are found in vegetable, corn, and soybean oil, soft margarine and butter, mayonnaise, nuts, and some cold water fish like salmon and tuna.

Portion Size: Amount of food eaten at one meal sitting.

Protein: Chains of amino acids which helps the body make muscle and grow.

Recommended Servings: The number of servings of foods (grains, fruit and vegetables, dairy products, and meats) for people of different ages, genders, and activity levels suggested by the USDA.

Refined Carbohydrates: Carbohydrates which are stripped of their fiber, vitamins, and minerals.

Regular Physical Activity: A pattern of exercise performed on a routine basis.

Salt: A mineral often used as a preservative of food and to season food. For some people, high salt diets can increase blood pressure.

Saturated Fats: Comes from animal sources, including meats and dairy products like whole milk, cheese, and ice cream, stick margarine, butter, and lard. These fats are easy to spot because they are solid at room temperature.

Serotonin: Often called the "feel good hormone" because it affects our moods and how we feel.

Simple Sugar: The smallest sugar possible. (For example glucose, but there are others.) Digested by the body very quickly.

Socioeconomic Status (SES): Refers to a person's level of income which allows him or her to afford housing, transportation, food, clothing, and other necessities.

Soluble Fiber: Fiber digestible by the body. It acts much in the same way a sponge absorbs water.

The Special Supplemental Nutrition Program for Women, Infants and Children (WIC): Assists women with children less than five years of age who cannot afford nutritious foods.

The Centers for Disease Control and Prevention (CDC): A federal agency that reports on disease and health statistics.

Trans Fats: Fats which are chemically manufactured from unsaturated fats by hydrogenation.

Triglycerides: A type of fat that the body normally stores and uses as a source of energy.

Unsaturated Fats: Liquid at room temperature. They come mainly from plant sources.

Vigorous-Intensity Physical Activity: Physical activity or exercise that requires a high level of effort in which a person experiences a large increase in breathing or heart rate. At this level of exercise, it is difficult to carry on a conversation. An example of this is running.

REFERENCES

American Academy of Pediatrics. Children, adolescents, and television. *Pediatrics*. 2001;107:423-426.

Baum CG, Forehand R. Social factors associated with adolescent obesity. *J Pediatr Psychol*. 1986;11:323-342.

Belamarich PF, Luder E, Kattan M, et al. Do obese inner-city children with asthma have more symptoms than nonobese children with asthma? Pediatrics. 2000;106 :1436–1441.

Bell NH, Shary J, Stevens J, Garza M, Gordon L, Edwards J. Demonstration that bone mass is greater in black than in white children. *J Bone Miner Res*. 1991;6:719–723.

Boutelle K, Neumark-Sztainer D, Story M, Resnick M. Weight control behaviors among obese, overweight, and nonoverweight adolescents. *J Pediatr Psychol*. 2002;27:531–540.

Bulik CM, Sullivan PF, Tozzi F, Furberg H, Lichetenstein P, Pederson NL. Prevalence, heritability, and prospective risk factors for anorexia nervosa. Arch Gen Psychiatry. 2006;63(3):305–312

Callahan ST, Mansfield MJ. Type II Diabetes Mellitus in adolescents. *Curr Opin Pediatr.* 2000;12:310–315.

Chobanian AV, Bakris GL, Black HR, et al. Seventh report of the Joint National Committee on Prevention, Detection, Evaluation, and Treatment of High Blood Pressure. *Hypertension.* 2003;42:1206–52.

Council on Sports Medicine and Fitness, Council on School Health. Active healthy living: prevention of childhood obesity through increased physical activity. *Pediatrics.* 2006;117:1834–1842.

Centers for Disease Control and Prevention. U.S. obesity trends 1985–2006. Centers for Disease Control and Prevention. *http://www.cdc.gov/nccdphp/dnpa/obesity/trend/maps/index.htm.* Updated July 27, 2007. Accessed January 5, 2008.

Centers for Disease Control and Prevention. 2005 YRBS results physical activity. Centers for Disease Control and Prevention.

CNN.com. No child left out of the dodgeball game? CNN.com. *http://www.cnn.com/2006/HEALTH/08/20/PE. NCLB/index.html.* Accessed January 15, 2008.

Crespo SJ, Smit E, Troiano RP, Bartlett SJ, Macera CA, Anderson RE. Television watching energy intake and obesity in US children. *Arch Pediatr Adolesc Med.* 2001;155:360–363.

Dietz WH, Gortmaker SL. Do we fatten our children at the television set? Obesity and television viewing in children and adolescents. *Pediatrics.* 1985;75:807–812.

The Expert Committee on the Diagnosis and Classification of Diabetes Mellitus. Follow-up report on the diagnosis of diabetes mellitus. *Diabetes Care.* 2003;26:3160–3167.

Freedman DS, Deitz WH, Srinivasan SR, Bao W, Newman WP. Association between multiple cardiovascular risk factors among children and adolescents: the Bogalusa Heart Study. *Pediatrics*. 1999; 103:1175–1182.

Harter S, Stocker C. The perceived directionality of the link between approval and self worth: the liabilities of a looking glass self orientation among adolescents. *J Adolesc*. 1996;6:285–308.

Hedley AA, Ogden CL, Johnson CL, Carroll MD, Curtin LR, Flegal KM. Overweight and obesity among US children, adolescents, and adults, 1999–2002. JAMA. 2004;291:2847–50.

Jahns L, Seiga-Riz AM, Popkin BM. The increasing prevalence of snacking among US children from 1977–1996. *Pediatrics*. 2001;138:493-498.

Janssen I., PhD, et al. Associations between overweight and obesity with bullying behaviors in school-aged children. *Pediatrics*. 2004;113:1187–1194.

Killian, Kyle D. (1994). Fearing fat: A literature review of family systems understandings and treatments of anorexia and bulimia. Family Relations, 43, 311–330.

Lambert, C. Ancient bodies collide with modern technology to produce a flabby, disease-ridden populace. *The Way We Eat Now*. 2004;106:50.

Lilenfield LR, Kaye WH. Genetic studies of anorexia and bulimia nervosa. In: Hock HW, Treasure JL, Katzman MA, eds. *Neurobiology in the Treatment of Eating Disorders*. Chichester: Wiley;1998:169–94.

Must A, Strauss RS. Risk and consequences of childhood and adolescent obesity. *Int Journal Obes Relat Metab Disord*. 1999;23(Suppl 2S2–S11).

National Association for Sport and Physical Education,
American Heart Association. *2006 Shape of the Nation
Report: Status of Physical Education in the USA*. Reston, VA:
National Association for Sport and Physical Education;
2006.

National Association of Anorexia Nervosa and Associated
Eating Disorders. *http://www.anad.org*. Accessed August 28,
2007.

National Center for Chronic Disease Prevention and Health
Promotion. Physical activity and health: a report of the
Surgeon General. *http://www.cdc.gov/nccdphp/sgr/adoles.htm*.
Accessed January 6, 2008.

National Center for Chronic Disease Prevention and Health
Promotion. Centers for Disease Control and Prevention.
*http://www.cdc.gov/diabetes/pubs/factsheets/
search.htm*. Updated December 20, 2005. Accessed
November 30, 2007.

National Center for Health Statistics. 2000 CDC growth
charts: United States. Centers for Disease Control and
Prevention. *http://www.cdc.gov/growthcharts/*. Accessed
January 5, 2008.

National Center for Health Statistics. Prevalence of overweight
among children and adolescents: United States, 1999–2002.
Centers for Disease Control and Prevention.
*http://www.cdc.gov/nchs/products/pubs/pubd/hestats/over-
wght99.htm*. Accessed January 5, 2008.

NIH Parents' Guide: National Cholesterol Education Program;
U.S. Department of Health and Human Services; National
Institute of Health, National Heart, Lung, and Blood
Institute, *NIH Publications*, No. 93–3102, September 1993.

Robinson TN, Chang JY, Haydel KF, Killen JD. Overweight concerns and body dissatisfaction among third-grade children: the impacts of ethnicity and socioeconomic status. *J Pediatr*. 2001;138:181–187.

Rushing JM, Jones LE, Carney C. Bulimia nervosa: a primary care review. *Prim Care Companion J Clin Psychiatry*. 2003;5(5):217–224.

Serrano, Elena. Preventing Childhood Obesity. *USDA Economic Research Service and the Farm Foundation*. April 2005. http://www.cdc.gov/HealthyYouth/physicalactivity/facts.htm <http://www.cdc.gov/HealthyYouth/physicalactivity/facts.htm> last accessed July 7, 2008.

Sorof JM, Lai D, Turner J, Poffenbarger T, Portman RJ. Overweight, ethnicity, and the prevalence of hypertension in school-aged children. *Pediatrics*. 2004;113;475–482.

Stephenson GD, Rose DP. Breast cancer and obesity: an update. *Nutr Cancer*. 2003;45(1):1–16.

Strauss P. Childhood obesity and self-esteem. *Pediatrics*. 2000;105: e15.

Sulti, L. The asthma obesity connection. *Am J Respir Crit Care Med*. 2005;171:659–64.

Tirodkar MA, Jain A. Food messages on African American television shows. *Am J Public Health*. 2003; volume 93 (3):439–441.

United States Department of Agriculture. *http://www.mypyramid.gov*. Accessed November 30, 2007.

US Department of Health and Human Services. *Healthy People 2010: Understanding and Improving Health*. 2nd ed. Washington, DC: US Department of Health and Human Services; 2001.

Vander Wal, JS, Thomas, N. Predictors of body image dissatisfaction and disturbed eating attitudes and behaviors in African American and Hispanic girls. *Eat Behav.* 2004;5:291–301.

Vaughn JL, King KA, Cottrell RR. Collegiate athletic trainers' confidence in helping females with eating disorders. *J Athl Train.* 2004;39(1):71–76.

Vestergarrd P, Emborg C, Stoving RK, et al. Fractures in patients with anorexia nervosa, bulimia nervosa, and other eating disorders: a nation wide register study. *Int J Eat Disord.* 2002;32:301–08.

Villiani S. Impact of media on children and adolescents: a 10–year review of the research. *J Am Acad Child Adolesc Psychiatry.* 2001;40(4):392–401.

Widerman MW, Pryor T. Substance use and impulsive behaviors among adolescents with eating disorders. *Addict Behav.* 1996;21(2):269–272.

Winkleby MA, Robinson TN, Sundquist J, Kraemer HC. Ethnic variation in cardiovascular disease risk factors among children and young adults. JAMA. 1999;281:1006–1013.

Zametkin AJ. Psychiatric aspects of child and adolescent obesity: a review of the past 10 years. *Focus 2004 2: 625–641.

ABOUT THE AUTHORS

Dr. Kathi A. Earles is presently the Medical Scientific Director for the Gulf region of Novo Nordisk, Inc. Prior to joining Novo Nordisk, she was the Assistant Director of the Morehouse School of Medicine (MSM) Pediatrics Residency program where she was instrumental in developing the curriculum and establishing the program from its inception. She continues to be an active faculty member at (MSM) where she participates in residency and graduate medical education and the Faculty Development Program at the MSM National Centers for Primary care.

Dr. Earles graduated from Howard University where she received a Bachelor of Science in Microbiology with a minor in Chemistry. After graduating from Howard University College of Medicine in 1991, she pursued a residency program at the University of Southern California in Los Angeles California. She later received a Masters in Public Health from the University of California/Los Angeles after which she assumed the position of Assistant Residency Program Director at Morehouse School of Medicine. She is a highly respected speaker, writer and educator on pediatric obesity and diabetes, and has a particular interest in the health disparities claiming the minority community. She was noted to be a Leading African-American Physician by *Black Enterprise* magazine in 2001 and has authored several publications including a chapter entitled "Epidemic on Overweight and Obesity" in *Health Disparities* with Dr. David Satcher, former Surgeon General.

Dr. Earles resides in Atlanta, Georgia where she deals most intimately with the struggles of keeping her own 3 children and husband healthy and active as well as those of the patients that she continues to serve.

Dr Sandra E. Moore is currently an Assistant Professor of Pediatrics at the Morehouse School of Medicine (MSM) in Atlanta, GA. Dr. Moore graduated cum laude from the University of Maryland Baltimore County (UMBC) in 1995 with a Bachelor of Science in Biochemistry and African American Studies. She received her Medical Degree form the University of Maryland Baltimore (UMAB) in 1999 and completed a Pediatric Internship and Residency at the University of Maryland Medical Center in 2002.

Dr. Moore joined the MSM faculty in July 2002. She completed Master of Science of Clinical Research (MSCR) at MSM in 2007. Dr. Moore has decided to devote her career to overweight in children. She has spoken at several conferences on this topic, including the National Medical Association (NMA) annual meeting in 2006. Her current research project examines maternal perception of children's weight. She recently presented the pilot study relating to this research at the 10th Research Centers in Minority Institutions (RCMI): International Symposium on Health Disparities. She has also authored several publications. She was awarded the National Institute of Health (NIH) Loan Repayment (LRP) based on her research.

The factor that drives Dr. Moore is her commitment to her patients. As a practicing community pediatrician, she is very much in touch with issues that affect her patients, and certainly the obesity epidemic is number one. She sees this struggle not only within her patients, but also within her colleagues, staff, peers, family, friends and self. This is why Dr. Moore decided to start an "overweight" clinic within the existing pediatric clinic in 2005, focusing on: 1) patient and family screening, counseling and follow -up 2) education of the staff and other physicians and 3) education and collaboration with the community.

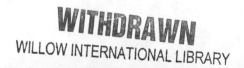